Life and Death

Life and Death

Moral Implications of Biotechnology

edited by

Viggo Mortensen

Published for the Lutheran World Federation by

WCC Publications, Geneva

Cover design: Edwin Hassink

ISBN 2-8254-1170-1

Printed in Switzerland

Contents

Preface

Bioethics is the term often used to describe the application of ethics to the biological sciences, medicine and related areas.

It seems sometimes that the findings of scientific research and the expanding possibilities for the technological exploitation of these discoveries are proceeding so rapidly that any concrete proposals for how they might be used responsibly are almost immediately obsolete. Yesterday's science fiction becomes today's scientific fact. There is an important relationship between Christian faith and these scientific and technological developments, because Christianity affirms that human beings are entrusted with life in order to be good stewards and to preserve the integrity of creation. The Christian belief in God as Creator and Redeemer includes a clear mandate of being responsible to God for one's own life, the lives of others and the created order as such. Christian bioethics must therefore try to discern what is God's will in all this and to reach a consensus with other opinions, both secular and religious.

In recent years the field of bioethics has developed greatly. Churches and their related research institutions have taken up bioethical issues simply because there has been quite a demand for them to do so. People are eager to hear what the church has to say — not necessarily in order to act accordingly, but at least in order to take what is said into account. But what can the church actually contribute?

The churches could try to develop an ethic which forms the basis for dialogue with people engaged in and affected by biotechnological developments. At the core of Christian ethics we do not find a list of ready-made answers but an invitation to reflect on controversial issues from the perspective of the biblical message and the Christian tradition. The stories Jesus told and the gospel record of his own life are resources which orient our thinking in a certain direction. The great commandment of love becomes the horizon against which we can reflect on bioethical issues in a way which is to the glory of God and the benefit of the neighbour.

Some churches have issued statements on bioethical issues. The value of these statements lies not only in their more or less favourable reception by various church bodies and institutions, but also in the process of reflection and debate underlying their drafting. It has been pointed out that discussions of bioethics have helped to turn the churches into communities of moral discourse.

With this publication the Lutheran World Federation would like to encourage this process. A working group nominated by the Nordic Lutheran churches reflected on how to stimulate reflection on bioethical issues; and this book is the result. The group felt it necessary first of all to outline clearly the basis from which it speaks. As we have said, bioethical questions confront all Christian churches. The foundation of our approach as a communion of Lutheran churches to this subject is set forth in the first chapter. Underlying it is our understanding of what it is to be a communion of churches. This notion of communion was adopted by the LWF eighth assembly in Curitiba in 1990. The various aspects of communion were described as follows:

- We see ourselves as a *spiritual* communion bound together in the Holy Spirit through our human faith in God our Father and Jesus Christ.
- We see ourselves as a *sacramental* communion, called by the gospel, united in baptism and gathered around the same table.
- We see ourselves as a *confessional* communion, grounded in scripture, the ecumenical creeds and the Lutheran confession.
- We see ourselves as a *witnessing* communion, cooperating and sharing interdependently with our Lutheran sisters and brothers and with other believers.
- We see ourselves as a *serving* communion, bearing the suffering and pain of others and serving as instruments of God's mercy and justice in the world.

In the first three points, communion is referred to as an already-existing reality grounded in God's ongoing work, nourished by the sacraments and founded in God's Word. A new understanding emerges in the last two points, which stress that full communion is not experienced unless it is translated into structures that promote cooperation, service and sharing. Using the notion of communion in a way that seeks to cover both doctrinal and ethical aspects is characteristic of the modern ecclesiological debate.

As a spiritual, sacramental, confessional, witnessing and serving communion, we stand in an intimate relationship to one another but are still struggling to define what that really means. The understanding I favour has its starting point in the communion table. To this table we come with all our differences, bound together by the Word of God. To this table we also bring the different gifts that have enriched our different traditions. The Lutheran tradition can therefore be seen as contributing to the wider ecumenical debate also in areas such as bioethics. This is the rationale behind our second chapter, which sets out resources for bioethics from the Lutheran tradition.

Having come this far, the group then analyzed how Luther did ethics. There are, of course, some relevant passages in his catechisms, but Luther did most of his social-ethical teaching in the form of letters and treatises written for specific occasions. The group therefore decided to do something similar. The remainder of this book then consists of eight imaginary letters written to different "players" on the bioethical scene. These letters are not meant to be read as authoritative statements by "experts" in ethics. When it comes to basic ethical questions there is no such thing as an expert. Rather, concerned Christians have, as a group, been reflecting on these issues from the perspective of the Christian message. In these letters feelings and sentiments are expressed and concrete information is given, so that readers might find it easier to make informed decisions on life-and-death issues arising in their own situation or that of people they know.

It is hoped that these "letters" can contribute in their own way to the building of a consensus. One of the most interesting features in ecumenical thought and activity is the underlying process. Naturally, the participants in these debates are always on the lookout for a possible agreement or consensus — with the risk that one is so eagerly seeking consensus that one gives up one's own identity. If that happens, the whole idea of seeking consensus loses its rationale. It is therefore of utmost importance to find the proper balance between consensus and identity in the ecumenical movement.

Bioethical issues often confront us with a variant of the same question. How does one reach an agreement, a consensus on whether a given procedure or technique is good or bad, right or wrong? What is the underlying premise? Is it possible to apply some of the insights gained ecumenically to the consensus-seeking process in contemporary bioethical thinking?

It is important that we consider the various religious traditions as a resource of knowledge and practical wisdom with regard to human life. The unique origin, value and purpose of human life continue to be fundamental themes in religious literature and life. Discussions of right and wrong, good and evil are inherent features of religious discourse.

Religious voices should be heard and respected in the discussion of the delicate and difficult moral issues associated with genetic research and counselling. Likewise, specifically religious perspectives should be tested in relation to other points of view. The beliefs and insights of all religious groups have a legitimate role in shaping public opinion and forming public policy. Diverse doctrines and commitments have a legitimate claim to be respected, heard, evaluated and applied in policy-making.

But although religious voices should be heard, the spectrum is broad; and if we are not to end up with a post-modern relativism like "I'm OK and you're OK", where everybody has a voice but nobody listens because nothing of any significance is being said, then we have to go one step further. The question then becomes one of how to say something from the very core of one's own tradition, in keeping with one's identity, while being open to a process whereby consensus is sought.

To conclude, I would like to thank not only all my fellow-contributors to this book but also Professor Paul Nelson (Wittenberg University, USA) and João Biehl (a doctoral student from Brazil), who especially helped us to focus our discussion at several points.

Viggo Mortensen

Part One

Bioethics and the Lutheran Communion

1. *What Is Bioethics?*

SVEIN AAGE CHRISTOFFERSEN

Peter and Paula are in love and would like to get married. But there is obviously a serious disease in Peter's family: several of his relatives have children with severe mental handicaps. What is the likelihood that children born to Peter and Paula will also have this disease? It is now possible for a medical examination to clarify this before they marry. Does Peter have a responsibility to accept such a pre-marital medical examination? Would it be right for Paula to leave him if the examination showed that some of his children would probably have the disease?

Sarah is pregnant and eagerly looking forward to being a mother. Then one day the doctor suggests an ultrasound scan to see if anything is wrong with the baby. If there is, Sarah can either choose to have an abortion or to continue the pregnancy. Is it right to offer an ultrasound scan on these terms? Is it right for Sarah to accept it?

Questions like these are often called "bioethical" questions. The word "bioethics" was coined in the late 1970s and has rapidly gained prominence in ethical debates in the 1980s and 1990s. The reason for this is its close connection to another fashionable word: "biotechnology". Bioethics is ethics with a special focus on challenges arising from modern biotechnology. To outline the significance of bioethics we therefore have to start with the significance of biotechnology.

Biotechnology may be defined as any technology using micro-organisms or biological material for technological purposes. Brewing is thus a form of biotechnology. In contemporary discussion, however, biotechnology is most closely associated with gene-technology. Gene-technology is a new kind of technology that seeks to alter the genes within a particular cell or group of cells. Genes are the building blocks of chromosomes, and the composition of chromosomes within a cell operates as a kind of programme to determine how a cell will grow and work. Thus by interfering in the genes we can in principle determine what is going on in the cell and how it will develop. Consequently, genetics and gene-technology incorporate a new kind of power over life and death.

If "biotechnology" is used to denote technology that either aims at altering the genes or draws on a certain amount of knowledge from modern genetics, the questions of bioethics then have to do in the broadest sense with the challenges raised by this new kind of power over life and death, especially in modern medicine. Adopting this broad sense of "biotechnology" and "bioethics", this chapter will address bioethical questions regarding human life at three different points: the beginning of life (prenatal medicine), in the midst of life (testing and screening) and at the end of life (euthanasia).

The beginning of life – prenatal medicine

Biotechnological possibilities of human interference with the beginning of life can be divided into two main groups: reproductive technology and prenatal diagnosis.

Reproductive technology. New technology now makes it possible to monitor, interfere with and to a certain degree even direct or control the reproductive process from the moment of fertilization. A human egg cell can be taken out of a woman, fertilized with sperm from her husband (or from another man) and afterwards put back into the woman's womb (or that of another woman). The main purpose of this technique, called in vitro fertilization (IVF), is to assist couples for whom it is difficult or impossible to have a baby of their own by normal sexual intercourse. This may be regarded as a good and respectable goal in itself. The wish to have a child of one's flesh and blood is deeply rooted in human nature. At the same time IVF creates new and hitherto unforeseen problems. Theoretically, a baby can now have three different mothers: the "genetic mother" (who provides the egg cell), the "surrogate mother" or "brooding mother" (who bears the baby within her body for nine months) and the "social mother" (who takes care of the baby after it is born). In most cases of IVF it is the same woman who provides the egg cell, carries the child within her and cares for it after birth, but IVF does make it possible for a woman to give birth to a baby that is not genetically her own or to act as a "brooding mother" for another woman.

Furthermore, an embryo produced in this way can be used for research rather than being placed in a woman's womb. An embryo can be kept alive outside the womb for approximately two weeks, and during this period it can be of great importance for modern medicine. But the embryo is at the same time a human being *in spe*, entitled to be handled with respect and care. Is it right to look at a human being *in spe* as just another object of research?

Prenatal diagnosis. Progress in medical technology has also made it possible to test babies before birth to detect abnormalities or complications. Information can be obtained on everything from its gender to deadly diseases. But little can be done to cure diseases that show up: in most cases the only two options for the woman are to have an abortion or to continue the pregnancy as before. An ultrasound scan is often the first step in detecting abnormalities. If it indicates that something is wrong, further tests are undertaken. Today, most pregnant women in many Western countries have an ultrasound scan during pregnancy.

In the midst of life – prospective tests and genetic screening

Modern medicine has also developed new ways of testing apparently healthy people for the probability of their becoming seriously ill in the future. Some diseases are completely determined by inheritance and difficult or impossible to avoid. Others result from the interplay between a person's gene-dispositions and his or her environmental influence or life-style. One may or may not become ill due to a whole array of different causes. These prospective tests can affect everyone, since we all are disposed to one disease or another; and screening programmes may be undertaken or offered to detect genetic defects on a large scale.

For some people information about possible future diseases will be of vital interest, enabling them to prepare for or even avoid a serious disease in advance. For others such information will create unnecessary anxiety or a false and perhaps dangerous feeling of security.

Healthy people may suddenly come to think of themselves as patients, while others may ignore sane and reasonable health precautions. Are we prepared and able to handle information like this in a good and balanced way? Still other people carry genes that will not affect their own health, but under certain circumstances may have consequences for the health of their children. They have no disease themselves, but if they conceive a child with a partner who has the same genetic defect, the child may become seriously ill. This possibility can now be clarified before marriage. Some will see this as vitally important; others may regard it as stigmatizing and wonder whether this is the first step towards requiring a kind of genetic certificate before marriage.

Knowledge is power; and recognizing that information from gene-tests will undoubtedly be of interest to insurance companies, employers and even democratic governments, many have raised their voices about the need to protect individuals from various forms of misuse of genetic information.

At the end of life – euthanasia

In itself the issue of euthanasia is not a consequence of new technological developments. Euthanasia — or mercy killing — has been discussed and debated for many centuries; it is dealt with, for example, in the Hippocratic oath. But for at least three reasons euthanasia has stimulated new discussions during the past ten to fifteen years.

One reason for this growing interest in euthanasia is the availability of new life-sustaining technologies. Contemporary techniques for keeping terminally ill patients alive have also created new possibilities of prolonging the death process. We are challenged in a new way to draw the line between meaningful life-sustaining treatment and the meaningless prolongation of a death process that only extends the pain and ignores the inevitability of death.

Another reason euthanasia has acquired a new interest, especially in Western countries, is the growing percentage of elderly people. This increasing number of frail and disabled elderly people has strained the ability of society to care for them. The weaknesses of old age have become more visible and urgent than before, and our ability to accept this weakness as a necessary part of life is apparently decreasing. Increasingly life has become unbearable for old and permanently ill people — and old people have increasingly become an intolerable burden on modern society. (The latter is perhaps a major reason for the former.)

A third reason for the interest in euthanasia today is probably that there is a new attitude towards life within modern societies. A meaningful and dignified life is associated with the ability of an individual to conduct his or her own life independently of others. To live is to take the opportunities that turn up and produce or consume as one wishes. Illness, disability and the need for care undermine one's self-respect and dignity in the eyes of others.

How does bioethics affect Christian communities?

Bioethical questions affect Christian communities in at least three different ways.

First of all, these issues touch the members of Christian communities in their daily lives as couples and families. In the years to come every pregnant woman, at least in Western societies, will be offered prenatal diagnosis of one form or another, and an ultrasound scan may become virtually universal. This means having to make decisions which have long-term consequences for daily life: to have a (more or less) disabled child or to have an abortion. For some, this will be the most important decision in their lives. And whatever they choose, they will have to live with the long-term consequences without a fixed answer to the question of right and wrong. They may regret their choices, but they will not be able to undo them. Some will appreciate having the opportunity to take such decisions; others will experience it as being forced to do the impossible.

Second, bioethical questions affect the members of the Christian communities as citizens. Politicians have to make laws and rules pertaining to how this new technology is to be used. As citizens, Christians have the civic duty to take part in the process of decision-making in their society. It may well be that the most important decisions determining what our societies will be like in the future are connected to these laws and regulations regarding biotechnology.

Third, members of Christian communities are involved in bioethical issues as part of a global church. It is within the power of this new technology to produce new kinds of injustice and exploitation between

North and South. Surely biotechnology will be used to help those who have the means to pay for it.

Multinational corporations are financing biotechnological research and development on a large scale. Big money is flowing into this industry, across national boundaries, and of course everybody wants to make their investments profitable. Thus biotechnology is being developed to help those people and societies who have money to pay for these kinds of services, and it will be designed to serve their interests and solve their problems. Few people in the third world will have the possibility to buy this technology. It will be available for the rich only.

This is not to say that the problems of wealthy nations and their affluent citizens are not real or serious problems. However, the point is that they will threaten to overrule the problems of the impoverished. When the biotechnological agenda is drawn up, problems concerning the third world are likely to be neglected. Research and development will be directed to serve interests in the North.

While new kinds of global injustice and exploitation arising from biotechnology may thus become visible within the one global Christian church, injustice is not an inevitable result of modern biotechnology. It may also be developed to help people in the third world. But this can happen only if people in the West are willing to pay for directing this kind of technology towards the needs of the poor, and to put the third world at the top of the agenda. Although this may seem like wishful thinking, it is the only possible way to avoid biotechnological development as just another widening of the gap between the rich and the poor. Every citizen in the Western world has a responsibility to speak on behalf of the poor in this situation, whether or not he or she is a Christian. But members of the Christian community should feel a particular urge to do so, because of the global perspectives within the Christian church itself.

The quest for ethics in a pluralistic society

Members of the Christian community have to face these issues within a pluralistic and in some ways post-modern society, characterized by moral fragmentation and polarization on the part of some and moral apathy on the part of others. In such a situation politicians may be tempted to reduce legislation concerning biotechnology to a minimum, leaving bioethical questions as far as possible to the individual's own choice. Two things are important to note in this connection.

First, we must realize that we cannot expect to solve all bioethical questions by legislation. We have to accept that in many cases people have the right to decide for themselves what is right and wrong. Society cannot make every decision for them. In this decision-making, however, the Christian community could offer considerable help, not only for Christians but also for people outside the Christian community. The Christian community should be able to help people to find an ethical foundation for their own decisions and to live with those decisions afterwards.

Second, even if not every question can find an answer through legislation, some questions can. Legislation is not everything, but it is at least something. Laws can establish a framework for ethical decisions and protect and secure human dignity; and the values that are basic to a just society set up barriers against dehumanizing forces in society. If we are to control multinational corporations by democracy, legislation is the only way. It is thus of vital importance to maintain the idea of just legislation determining the kind of society we are heading for. Without some kind of legislative control over developments in the field of biotechnology, it will be impossible to solve the conflicts between the Western and the developing world.

In this situation the Christian community must insist on the idea of a common and reasonable ethical foundation for common legislation in spite of moral fragmentation and apathy. Pluralism can be a temptation to the church, because it can be used as an excuse to withdraw from the public exchange of different views into an ethical discourse meant only for Christians. Rather, the church, and not least the Lutheran church, should be a community of moral discourse common to all people.

2. *The Lutheran Approach to Bioethics*

LARS ØSTNOR, JAANA HALLAMAA,
SVEND ANDERSEN, BJÖRN BJÖRNSSON,
GERT NILSSON and LARS THUNBERG

The purpose of this chapter is to reflect on bioethical questions on the basis of the Lutheran theological heritage. In doing so we will draw on positions marked by Luther himself, but primarily on the Lutheran doctrinal tradition and the views of Lutheran churches today.

For Luther and the subsequent Lutheran tradition, it is characteristic that ethical standpoints have a religious basis of the theocentric kind: their foundation is the work and will of the triune God. This implies that ethical knowledge and moral life must be seen in association with the proclamation of God's acts and with people's belief.

All people are created by God and have their continued existence by virtue of the sustaining work of the Creator. As recipients of life and of the benefits of creation, all human beings are responsible to God, whether or not they confess any faith. Therefore, everyone has to account to God for how he or she has used the gifts of creation. Against this background Christian ethics, including bioethics, according to a Lutheran point of view, addresses all individuals and collective groups. Such an ethic intends to express the demands to which all of us as creatures are subject.

God's action in history in his Son Jesus Christ and his ongoing work through the Holy Spirit for the salvation of human beings and the whole world give another foundation to ethical commandments: we who are so greatly loved by the Saviour are bound to live in love towards each other. At this level Christian ethics is able to address the faithful from the background of a specific presupposition and unique motivation.

Created in God's image, fallen into sin

One way of bringing out what lies behind different ethical issues is to observe that questions like "Who am I?" or "What is it to live a human life?" express a fundamental concern common to our ethical dilemmas. Such questions can be answered at different levels. For example, human beings are all members of a biological species; they can thus be scrutinized from a biological point of view. Or human life can be described using the perspectives offered by anthropological research. While both biological and anthropological knowledge are relevant for determining the nature of human life, however, such knowledge is not enough for establishing an answer when we ask ethical questions. Moral questions deal not only with factual knowledge and information about how the world is, but also with values and norms. Finding an answer to fundamental moral questions means determining what makes our lives meaningful and valuable and what strengthens or threatens our integrity and well-being.

In the following, we ask what the Lutheran tradition and Lutheran theological ethics have to offer for people confronted with bioethical problems. In doing so, we shall use language and deal with questions which may often seem remote from the concrete and practical moral dilemmas we face in biomedicine. Nevertheless, there are two reasons why this use of language is meaningful here. First, in Lutheran theology, as in all Christian theology, questions like "Who am I?" and "What is human life?" cannot be answered without referring to God, the ground and source of all being. Second, the basic relation human beings have to God cannot be expressed without using religious language, and one cannot translate this language into other modes of speech without losing something essential.

In the Christian understanding of reality, God is the beginning and end of everything, the source and aim of all existence, the creator and sustainer of all there is. Without God nothing comes into existence and without God's sustaining power nothing can stay alive or continue to exist. Everything in the universe owes its being to God. From this perspective, the most fundamental question to anything that exists is its relation to God. To ask what it is to be a human being in general or what it is to be a particular human being means, then, to ask what our relationship is to God.

The Bible describes the essential relationship of the human being to God by saying that God has created the human being in God's image (*imago Dei*) to be man and woman. To understand human life in these terms is to acknowledge that human beings are radically dependent in three ways: our life depends on God, on God's creation, the universe, and on other people. Of these three the first is of fundamental meaning and importance because our relationship to God determines the two other relationships: if our relation to God is distorted, it necessarily affects our relation to other people and to the created world. According to the Christian understanding, Jesus Christ is the image of true humanity, in whom we see both the original nature of God's image and its fulfillment.

Being created in God's image involves basically two things: a gift and a task. The heart of this gift is a special relationship in which God freely and abundantly shares his goods — love, goodness, beauty, wisdom — with human beings. The task implied by being created in the image of God is to become God's co-workers, stewards and cultivators of the earth.

These two aspects of the *imago Dei* are combined in the fact that human beings are moral beings. This means that they are responsible agents who are accountable for their deeds and works, primarily to God and secondarily to each other. Moral accountability is a specifically human characteristic in the sense that being morally responsible differentiates human beings from both angels and animals. At the first instant of their being, angels determine the direction of their will — either towards God and his will or against God and towards the will of God's adversary. Angels are responsible only for this first choice, which determines all their subsequent actions; and in this sense they do not belong to the sphere of morality. Animals, for their part, belong to the moral realm only as objects of moral concern and not as moral subjects, for they are completely unaccountable for their deeds and cannot be punished or reproached for anything they do. Human beings are different. Being created in God's image originally means a freedom to choose, a freedom to will and, for this reason, moral responsibility.

Human beings are only a very small part of God's creation. The task of cultivating and keeping given to human beings does not mean that they are set to be rulers or exploiters of the creation. The total dependence of bodily human life on nature and on its flourishing manifests this. Human beings share the destiny of the rest of the creation, its well-being as well as its destruction.

The biblical story of the creation involves human life taking bodily form as a sexual being, as a man or as a woman. The theological meaning of this is that no human being comes to life without having parents and without being born from another human being. In addition, no one can become a human person outside the human community. Consequently, the ideal of an independent, self-sufficient life has no point or meaning. Human life is essentially dependent on other human beings.

These three dependencies and relationships form the absolute determinants of human life according to the Lutheran understanding, and they establish the starting point for ethics. The implications of this understanding are both normative and theoretical. Belief in God as the source and sustainer of everything that exists makes human life an absolute gift, whose quality and worth are independent of all human attempts to evaluate it. From this perspective, human life is an end in itself. It has intrinsic value irrespective of whose life it is and of what kind of life it is. No one deserves the God-given worth and dignity of life, and no one can be deprived of it by anything or by anyone. As part of the created world, human beings may not use their abilities and capacities to exploit nature or to degrade it into a mere means for purely human ends. Membership of the human community makes people dependent on each other but it also points to the call to human beings to live in mutual support, to a life in which the whole community is responsible for the good of its individual members.

In addition to these normative implications, creation has theoretical importance for the Lutheran understanding of ethics. Being created by God means that every human being is an image of God and must be treated accordingly. Furthermore, all people are moral agents and ethical subjects morally responsible to God and to each other. This conviction can also be expressed by saying that by virtue of God's creation human beings share the natural moral law. As an *imago Dei* every human being has a conscience, that is, a natural understanding of good and evil and the difference between them. But the existence of this natural moral law which all people share simply because they are human beings is not a claim about empirical reality: Lutheran ethics does not maintain that all people actually share a similar understanding of right and wrong. The idea of natural law expresses the belief that all human beings have moral dignity and a conscience, whose voice must be respected. This makes possible discussion of and co-operation in moral questions regardless of people's religious or political convictions and opinions. Human beings share the same status as being created in God's image, and for this reason they must be treated as responsible and autonomous subjects.

This harmonious picture of the human being created in the image of God and living in a perfectly good relationship to God, nature and other people does not of course correspond with reality. Our personal experience and the lives of other people attest to broken relations, hatred instead of love, cruelty where there should be tenderness, evil replacing the good. This reality reflects what in religious language is called sin. Instead of being open to God the source of life, to the needs of other creatures and to community with other people, human beings have turned in on themselves (*incurvatus/a in se*). The essence of sin is this distorted self-concentration and self-sufficiency, the will to be one's own sole aim and end. From this distorted direction of one's will arise all evil thoughts and deeds.

Sin is a basic perversion which stains everything that human beings are and do. It affects the way they see God, the creation, other people and themselves. It also has an impact on their conception of good and evil. For this reason, all human ethical thinking is necessarily defective. Still, human beings are aware of the fundamental difference between right and wrong, even if they cannot discern it clearly in a particular situation. They feel themselves called to do good and to avoid evil. However, in a world existing under the conditions of sin, even the best deeds are inevitably corrupted by it and by its distorting effects.

Justification

Ethics as the consideration of what is the right way to act towards other human beings cannot stand alone. In the language of the Lutheran tradition, ethics has a limited perspective, in that it deals with things *coram hominibus* (in relation to human beings). This perspective must always be connected with another one, which is –

again in the traditional language — *coram Deo* (in relation to God). Ethics must, as stressed above, always be seen in connection with our relation to God.

What should this relation be? Traditionally, the same words are used for the relation to God as for relations among human beings. One central word is "just". Human beings have to be just to God or do justice to God. Luther's thinking on justice was inspired by the concept of justice common in his day, which defined it as giving to everyone his due (*suum cuique*). What should we give to God? We should recognize God as the one he is: our good creator.

We might try to do justice to God by doing good deeds, that is, by trying to live up to what we think God expects of us. To have this attitude is to suppose that God demands from us a kind of achievement, and if we succeed we do God justice and deserve his love.

In thinking this way, we relate ourselves to God by way of the law. In a way, this is as it should be. The law is the expression of God's will, and what we have just talked about — doing justice to God — is the content of the first of the Ten Commandments. Nevertheless, by trying to attain a right relation to God through our own achievement, we demonstrate that this relationship is in a state of disorder. We have to acknowledge that we cannot achieve what we think the law demands. To come back to the vocabulary of the tradition, we are confronted by the law in its second use, the spiritual or theological. When we use the law as prescribing achievements by which we hope to deserve the love of God, the law shows us that what it demands — primarily recognition of God — cannot be obtained by achievement. The law thus reveals that we cannot come by our own power into a right relationship towards God. We cannot do him justice. The law becomes God's condemning speech to us: "You *shall*, but you *cannot*!"

But functioning this way, the law prepares us to hear quite a different speech from God, namely the gospel. The gospel is the word that what we seek to obtain by achievement is given to us. What we cannot do — justice to God — Jesus Christ has done on our behalf. The content of the gospel is that God offers us a share in the justice of Christ. The offer is without conditions; we do not have to achieve anything first, we just have to accept the offer. The acceptance of the offer is what happens when we have faith, that is, trust that we share in the justice of Christ and thus stand as just before God ourselves.

There is a danger that this idea of justification can become a "doctrine" which we grasp intellectually but which does not move us as living human beings. Thus we must make it clear that the particular words "justification" and "just" are not necessarily the crucial thing. As we have seen, Luther used the term "justice" against the background of the understanding of his time. Today, "justice" is often used with quite different meanings. This is one of the reasons we must seek the core behind the doctrine and concepts. The core is that we cannot live our life as given by a loving Creator if we make our own achievement the most important thing and that it is Jesus of Nazareth who by his life and death reconciles us with God our Father and shows us what a life given by a loving Creator is like. Belief in resurrection is the belief that the life and work of Jesus is the true expression of the love of the Creator. Faith in Christ is the acquisition of his life and grace in such a way that it makes us "a new creation". In faith, we live our life out of a creating power which wishes us well. We have acquired the right relationship to God and have the right attitude towards our life. We are "justified".

This does not mean that sin has totally disappeared. We are justified in the sense that God counts us as just; and our believing this makes it possible to have the right attitude towards God and our own life. But sin is still there, inciting us to do evil. To be a Christian, then, is to be just and sinner at the same time (*simul justus et peccator*).

Neighbourly love

When we as believers have this attitude towards our life, we regard it as manifestation of a good act, both by Christ and by God. Christ has acted on our behalf. He has restored our distorted relationship to God. We are thereby able to see our life in the right light — as a gift from our good Creator. Faith means that we understand ourselves as beings who were in need and who were helped. In faith we see that we are objects of love. God and Christ have placed themselves in our position and unselfishly acted to our best.

Therefore, faith can manifest itself in joy, the joy of gratitude. In our view, this joy cannot be kept within the closet of our own inner life or closed within the sanctuary of the church. The joy of faith is directed towards God (*coram Deo*), but it also turns our sight towards our fellow creatures, in the first place our fellow human beings (*coram hominibus*). And our view towards our fellow human beings is coloured by the thought that "as I was object of God's goodness and care, I want to show care towards human beings who need it". In other words, faith contains the thought, "I want to love my neighbour as I was loved myself". This thought is not a consciousness of duty. It is inseparably linked with the very joy of faith. If faith is really present, it cannot help manifesting itself in an active effort to serve our neighbour. Faith is liberation from the enforcement of achievement, which is why we can let our good deeds be exclusively directed towards our fellow human being.

Luther often summed up the content of neighbourly love in two words: beneficence and suffering. While the first seems obvious, many might wonder why suffering is part of neighbourly love. Some have even accused Christians of a kind of masochism — seeking suffering for its own sake. Neighbourly love as the manifestation of faith is unselfish. The believer places himself or herself in the position of the other and does what serves the other. Thus the believer can neglect his or her own wishes, desires and interests or give them lower priority in case of conflict with the interests of others. It would be hypocritical to claim that we can be unselfish in this sense without implying suffering.

But how can the believer be prepared for that suffering? One could answer that belief or faith itself contains suffering. If faith is acquisition of the life of Jesus Christ — a life which by suffering reconciled us with God — then the joy of faith can only be the kind of joy which you cannot have without suffering. And as we cannot receive the love of God without suffering, we cannot pass it on in the shape of neighbourly love without suffering.

What we have just said is expressed in the tradition in terms of the close connection between the two perspectives *coram Deo* and *coram hominibus*. In the New Testament this connection is expressed by the double commandment of love: "You shall love the Lord your God with all your heart, and with all your soul, and with all your mind... You shall love your neighbour as yourself" (Matthew 22:37,39). Still another way of expressing this connection is to say that the gospel, the faith and the foundation of neighbourly love are spiritual. They are manifestations of God's spiritual kingdom. That means, among other things, that they involve a way of acting which does not depend on force and coercion. But this kingdom of God is not only an inner entity. The acts of God in this kingdom can only be received in freedom. And the subject of this free reception can only be an individual human being. But the spiritual is also a kingdom in the sense of a community of believers, whose external and visible sign is the church, the people gathered around the Word and the sacraments (we shall come back to its contemporary role later). As a contrast to this kingdom stands the worldly one, where God sometimes acts by external force — the so-called first use of the law, the enforcement of norms by sanctions such as punishment.

The Christian in the world

We must confess that our churches have often presented the distinction between these two kingdoms in a way which suggests that both faith and neighbourly love are exclusively something inner and invisible, of which only the individual could be aware. In our view, this presentation is a misunderstanding. We must therefore say something about the third aspect of Christian life: *coram mundo* (in relation to the world).

The world (*mundus*) is where the common life of human beings takes place without necessarily being dominated by faith and the spiritual. It is where Satan, the adversary of God, plays his games, and where human acts are coloured by sin, that is, the distorted relationship to God. The character sin gives to human acts is evil. When a human being does not regard his or her life as the manifestation of a good or loving act, he or she is not necessarily motivated to do good to other human beings.

The world, however, is not left by God. On the contrary, God also acts in the world. God has a worldly kingdom, and God's maintenance of it consists in his repressing the destruction of sin and evil by external means. Among these means is the law, as we have already mentioned. The law and the juridical system must be maintained by political authority, for which Luther normally uses the term "prince" (king or emperor). Persons in authority are not just individuals who have obtained political power. They are holders of an office which is instituted by God. The office is part of the order by which the Creator represses his adversary. Besides the political offices (*politia*) Luther also considers the roles of the household (*oeconomia*), primarily that of the father, as an order created by God.

But God does not act in the world only as a protecting agency against evil. Such protection presupposes that there is something to be protected — which is created human life and fellowship among human beings in family and society. Human life and community are good things which require certain external conditions if they are to flourish, first of all peace and some material resources. As Creator, God is the origin of the good human life and his orders thus serve the positive goal of forming a framework within which the good human life and community are realized.

On this understanding, the world is also the place where Christians practise neighbourly love. We should note in particular several of the claims Luther makes regarding the relation of the Christian to the worldly:

(1) The Christian can recognize such worldly orders as political authority and marriage as manifestations of God's good acts of creation. Christians must therefore support these orders and not contribute to the discredit of the worldly by turning their backs on it.

(2) The character of suffering of neighbourly love means that the Christian does not necessarily make use of the worldly orders — such as the judicial system — to his or her own advantage. On the contrary, the Christian is prepared to refrain and to suffer injustice, provided that it is only his or her own interests that are at stake ("Do not resist an evildoer. But if anyone strikes you on the right cheek, turn the other also; and if anyone wants to sue you and take your coat, give your cloak as well"; Matthew 5:39-40).

(3) If, on the other hand, a fellow human being is involved, neighbourly love as beneficence has the effect that the Christian will make use of the worldly orders to the benefit of the other.

(4) One way of using the worldly as a means of showing neighbourly love is to hold a worldly office. For example, a Christian may be "prince". If so, that person must use this worldly power — political, juridical, economic, military — not to his or her own benefit but to that of the subjects. Having a worldly office is one

way of fulfilling a calling, that is, living up to the demands inherent in the social roles one plays.

(5) Because the world is marked by God's creative goodness, no human being is totally without knowledge of the good and of the right way of acting. Every human being knows by his or her reason what traditional terminology called the natural law. Only the believer, it is true, shows unselfish neighbour-love out of gratitude for the gift of Christ. But because Christians can see the world as God's creation, they can presuppose that non-Christians also have a knowledge of the natural law. To Luther, natural law is summarized in the Golden Rule: "In everything do to others as you would have them do to you" (Matthew 7:12).

We should not ignore the fact that Luther's view of the worldly was shaped and limited by the conditions of his time. Otherwise there is a risk that the Lutheran understanding of Christian faith becomes a legitimation of feudal and other authoritarian power structures. At the same time, recognizing the time-relatedness of Luther's ideas of the worldly should not lead to a total rejection of them. The distinction between the spiritual and the worldly is essential to our understanding of Christian faith, but if we want to retain it, we are obliged to take into account that the worldly in our days is something different from what it was at the time of the Reformation.

What Luther calls the "worldly" corresponds to what we mean today when we talk about the social and the political, that is, the public framework within which people live their common life. In our opinion, Christians should recognize the following facts and viewpoints about modern societies:

(a) The best way of political organization is generally taken to be democracy. Thus we cannot operate with a division of people into subjects and sovereigns. Every citizen in a democratic state is sovereign and subject at the same time.

(b) Modern societies are dynamic. There are no immutable external orders or institutional frameworks; on the contrary, they often change.

(c) Institutions in a modern society are neither established from eternity nor a result of contingent happenings. Institutions are created by human beings.

(d) Modern society is not just one country or continent or empire, but the whole community of humankind. The "worldly" of today is global.

Because the world of today looks different in these ways from the worldly of Luther's time, the realization of neighbourly love must have a different shape. But the principal point is the same: the world is, as well as the church, the place where Christians act in the best interest of their fellow human beings. Let us now try to sketch the contemporary shape of neighbourly love in society.

First of all, neighbourly love points to a democratic organization of the political order. That is because neighbourly love does not only mean beneficence, but also equality: in the light of Christian faith, every human life is of equal importance. This fundamental equality does not mean that all human beings are to be treated the same way in each and every respect; indeed, to do so would mean that many people were treated unlovingly. But equality means at least that every differential treatment must be given a valid justification. And there is no justification for treating adult people unequally in regard to participation in political power.

A principal task for Christians is thus to contribute to the establishment and maintenance of democratic societies. Next, they should use their power to organize societies so that they accord as far as possible with the principles of beneficence and equality contained in neighbourly love. Together these two principles entail that all human beings are entitled to a just share of the goods at hand, not just to help in the form of charity. The unity of beneficence and equality entails justice, and justice means among other things that the goods — the prerequisites for leading a decent and perhaps happy life — are distributed with equality as an ideal. Whereas it is evidently utopian to suppose that this ideal could be realized in the shape of total equality, it does involve the demand that every inequality must be justifiable.

An important consequence of the distinction between the two kingdoms is that worldly power does not have access to the belief of the individual. In Luther's time, this was the foundation that entitled the Christian to claim non-interference by political authority in questions of belief. In the democratic societies of our day Christians should extend this idea in two directions. First, we must say that this freedom also applies to believers of other religions. Second, we must understand it as more than freedom of religious belief. A democratic society must allow space for every human being to shape his or her life — in his own way, on her own accountability. In this sense, democracy cannot work without liberty. But the space of freedom is demarcated by the framework of the orders defined by the other principles of neighbourly love: beneficence, equality and justice.

In seeking to realize these principles within the framework of democracy, Christians enter the open dialogue about the principles of organizing institutions which is a necessary part of democracy. In this dialogue, they meet people who do not share their religious starting point. Nevertheless, Christians can presuppose that their dialogue-partners are acquainted with the natural counterpart of neighbourly love: the Golden Rule. On the one hand, this rule must be interpreted within a church tradition as a principle summarizing the substance of Christian ethics and as part of the proclamation of Jesus (cf. Matthew 7:12). On the other hand, the Golden Rule may be understood as a singular ethical norm belonging to various religions and cultures, using related formulations. Thus, we should not regard ourselves as just another community with just one of a multitude of particular moral systems. We can regard the principles of neighbourly love as something which by being transferred to the worldly order can form part of a moral consensus. But we must keep in mind that this kind of ethics is not necessarily the same as the way of life the individual Christian chooses for himself or herself on the basis of his or her own faith.

Christian ethics, then, in our understanding, has two elements. One has to do with the consequences individual Christians draw from their faith for their own life: they must decide in each situation how to realize unselfish and suffering "Christ-life" personally and in their vocation. The other element is the effort by Christians to transfer neighbourly love to the worldly sphere and thus to contribute to organizing a social order on the basis of the principles of beneficence, equality, justice and liberty. This realization of neighbourly love entails, perhaps paradoxically, that Christians leave space to non-Christians to lead their life in ways quite different from the way Christians have chosen for themselves.

Culture and Scripture

Cultural elements. Both human beings and institutions in society are responsible to God as creator and saviour when they make decisions on ethical questions, including bioethical ones. But what enables them to take this responsibility seriously?

According to Lutheran tradition, the life-conditions of human beings in the moral field are decisively determined by the existence of a universal ethical knowledge, the so-called natural law (*lex naturalis*). "Natural" in this context indicates that this knowledge belongs to everybody by virtue of creation: that is, the rational potential of the human being and his or her belonging to a social context which is placed under the laws of the Creator.

Natural law manifests itself in several ways: in reason, in life-experience and in the conscience of human beings. But this should not be seen in a purely individualistic way. Natural law includes the collective understanding of a group or a society of what is reasonable and the wisdom of their common life.

As regulator of behaviour, natural law is not to be identified with abstract inborn ideas in human consciousness. It is something historical which asserts itself in relations between humans and in a person's relation to himself or herself and to nature. Here it confronts us with demands that emerge from the reality of life around us, of which we ourselves are a part. Theologically interpreted, these demands express God's ongoing work as creator in the world. Quite apart from whether or not the individual acknowledges the moral demands as divine commandments, natural law provides conditions for ethical insights and moral life among people in general.

Paul speaks in Romans 2:14f. of the presence of this moral consciousness among those who do not have the law as revealed in the Jewish-Christian history of salvation. He concentrates on the content of "what the Law requires", which everyone can recognize, and disregards the different frameworks of faith or religion in which the law can be placed. Luther speaks in a similar way when he talks about how human beings are subject to natural law in political and social questions, irrespective of their religion and view of life.

In the Lutheran tradition the content of natural law has been defined by central moral-normative passages in the Old and New Testaments. The natural law is equivalent to the Decalogue (Exodus

20:1-17), or to the double commandment of love towards God and our neighbour (Matthew 22:34-40) or to the commandment of love towards our neighbour (Leviticus 19:18; Matthew 22:39; Romans 13:8f.; Galatians 5:14), or to the Golden Rule (Matthew 7:12; Luke 6:31). Natural law is thus to be interpreted as a demand for faith and for acts of love within the family bond and the professional, political and other relations in which we live.

Historically, the concept of natural law has expressed a central theological concern. However, if it is to be used fruitfully in our time, it is necessary to avoid the tendencies to abstract, unhistorical rationalism and individualism and reconstruct the concept by seeing the human being in a context of fellowship and society and against the background of an historical tradition. We prefer therefore to speak of the normative, moral aspects of the culture, referring to the ideas, values, norms and symbols that are transferred — as a rule with some changes — from generation to generation, and to the social structures in which they appear. This is not to deny that a given cultural tradition may comprise contrasts and differing factors; still, the values and symbols of a culture include normative-ethical elements which establish uniting patterns in society and support and undergird individuals and societies in a constructive way. Some of these ethical norms are shared across the borders of societies and cultures.

Such moral factors in the culture also provide premises for practical cooperation between Christians and non-Christians in ethical concerns, for instance those of modern bioethics.

Scripture alone. But to what extent can the content of common moral elements in cultural traditions provide a sufficient and valid basis for the discussion of bioethical issues?

Lutheran theology has a two-sided evaluation of the potential of natural law. On the one hand, from the perspective given by belief in creation, Lutherans accept the possibility of making personal choices and establishing structures in society which correspond to the commandment to love our neighbour. On the other hand, they recognize that the conditions for proper conduct of life and commonality of values in society are corrupted. This dual approach reflects the evaluation of contemporary morals in biblical texts, which combine a "yes" to some aspects of the existing behaviour and systems with a "no" to morally critical conditions (cf. Philippians 4:8; Romans 13:

1-5; Ephesians 4:17-24; Colossians 3:5-8). The former is supported by belief in creation, the latter by awareness of the fall and the consequences of sin on the moral level.

The fall has consequences for both ethical knowledge and discernment — a complete and adequate insight into the content of God's law — and practical moral living — the ability to live according to it. Paul unfolds this viewpoint in Romans 1:19ff. and 3:9ff. Against this background Luther, and the Lutheran churches following him, have operated with Scripture as a corrective also in moral questions. Scripture can have this function because it is the witness to the historic revelation of God's will, as mediated through Moses and the prophets in the Old Covenant and through Jesus and the apostles in the New Covenant.

Historically the normativity of the Scripture has often been expressed theologically by the formula "Scripture alone" (*sola scriptura*). While this principle is taken to apply to the complete doctrinal content of the Christian message, both law and gospel, opinions differ within Lutheran churches and among Lutheran theologians about how it is to be understood with reference to actual ethical problems. Tentatively, the following directions can be noted:

(1) The role of Scripture as a source for ethical knowledge supplements but does not eliminate the sources given by virtue of the universal revelation to all human beings (reason, life experience, conscience). In societies within the Christian tradition, Scripture is itself part of the cultural heritage. At the same time, it transcends all human realities: through these particular texts God speaks to individuals and societies.

(2) As the witness of the revelation of God's moral law within history, the Bible has a specific authority as the word of God. With regard to ethical problems, this means that special attention must be given to arguments based on norms or perspectives which are substantial parts of the biblical texts (for example, theological anthropology, the doctrine of nature and history, the Decalogue).

(3) This does not ascribe general authority to each ethical statement in Scripture. It is the Bible as a whole that is the normative source for knowledge. Each different passage is to be read in its textual and historical context. The use of the Bible in ethics presupposes a hermeneutical task, a work of interpretation in which the details

are seen in the light of the totality and the periphery is differentiated from the centre — the message about Jesus Christ, his person, work and will. At the same time, the differences of social, economic and political context between the time of the Bible and the present must be taken into account. On the basis of such a reflection, theology has to offer criteria for the legitimate use of the Scripture in ethics.

References to biblical texts in discussions of ethical problems are valid not only within theology and the church. As a classical text with a long and pervasive influence in certain cultural traditions, Scripture also has relevance for the debate within society about bioethics and other difficult moral problems.

Ecumenical perspectives. The Lutheran churches share with other churches the conviction that the Christian community has important contributions to make to the ethical debate of our time. The churches do not enter this debate claiming to have definitive solutions to these problems, but in order to make their specific contributions to the ongoing clarification of issues. Their voice in this field combines ordinary argumentation using different types of good reasons with a unique proclamation presenting the Christian worldview and anthropology and biblical norms.

Within the Christian community the Lutheran church will be particularly engaged in two ways. Over against all exclusively biblically related conceptions, Lutherans will stress the existence of natural law and the fact that individuals belong to a social and historical culture with normative elements. Over against a one-sided emphasis on the capacity of human reason and the importance of the cultural aspect, they will point to the need to supplement these with the texts of the Bible, giving the ethos of the particular revelation. The specific Lutheran contribution to Christian ethics is thus a certain combination of different perspectives: a positive evaluation of the dimension of creation, leading to an acceptance of natural law and normative, cultural ideas, a realistic understanding of the ethical deprivation resulting from the fall and a focus on the definite disclosure of God's ethical will mediated to us through Scripture.

Sharing certain cultural elements with all people "of good will", Lutherans participate in the ethical dialogue in society. Having the

Bible as a treasure in common with all Christianity, they are open to dialogue with other churches.

Bioethics, the church and the last things

The role of the church in social ethics. One often hears it said that the task of the church is to preach the gospel and administer the sacraments, not to deal with matters of science, technology, economics and so on, which are the province of specialists and politicians. This probably explains why ethics and especially social ethics are rarely found on the agenda of important concerns in many churches. The churches give their attention to spiritual matters. Politicians and specialists run the world, and churches are unable to address questions about social and political life.

This is a wrong interpretation of the doctrine of the two kingdoms. According to the theology of Martin Luther, God is the king of the two kingdoms. We are not permitted to separate one part of reality and exempt the Christian church from responsibility for it.

But what is the church? In the Lutheran tradition, the church is not a political institution but a spiritual one, a movement and a community. The church expresses itself by preaching the gospel and distributing the sacraments, by educating and pastoral counselling, and in the daily life of believers. Participating in the ethical debate is a task primarily for Christian preaching and education rather than for bishops and synods. The foundation of the ethical decisions in the church is theology, not politics. Of course, the church is also an institution. Its task is to serve the gospel on its way to all people, not to be a ruler over it. All members of the church have to live as Christians in their daily life and so express their Christian faith.

This means that the Christian view of bioethics, for example, cannot be decided by church leaders alone. Rather, it must be formulated in a discourse among church leaders, theologians, pastors, scientists and parishioners.

Moreover, since the church is a movement, not a static institution, the temporary character of Christian ethics must be recognized. The problems it addresses are continually changing; they differ from one place to another and from one time to another.

Sending out his disciples, Jesus gave them a twofold mission: to preach the gospel and to cure sick people. The church has often emphasized the first part of this twofold mission while tending to neglect the second. This neglect has had serious consequences for the church and human beings. If the church is to be faithful to its twofold mission today, it must involve itself in such contemporary issues as technology, biotechnology and medicine. But the church does not have a monopoly in the area of ethics. Moreover, the church's main task is to proclaim the gospel of forgiveness of sins and to encourage people to live; and its ethical proclamation must conform with this mission.

The Lutheran view of the church is not easy to formulate. It is a third way between institutionalism and individualism. The church is a community of Christian believers, and this community is united by the living word of God, baptism and the eucharist. Moral decisions are not grounded in authoritative utterances from the institution nor in purely individual intuition; instead, discourse on ethical matters is something that must be going on continuously.

As moral responsibility moves from the private to the public level, it moves simultaneously from the individual Christian believer to the church. The social responsibility of the church is to witness before the world, *coram mundo*, about human dignity and human rights on the basis of the fundamental relationship between the human being and God. The church itself is called to be a community of people which makes visible this primary relationship of love and justice in its life as a fellowship. To the extent that the church is faithful in executing this calling, it will fulfill the most important part of its moral obligation. The ultimate moral responsibility of the church is to be the church.

In fulfilling this calling, the church is commissioned also to address the public authorities, invoking their moral responsibility as custodians of law and justice.

At the broadest level of society and public responsibility, more and more bioethical issues focus on the question of legislation. Thus the question of what are the duties and responsibilities of the state and legislative bodies must be taken into critical consideration.

Should the church give moral directions to legislation? According to Lutheran theology, the church has to bring up to date inviolable values founded on the Christian view of creation and human beings. On the basis of a vision of the good life, the church must show how society may be better. But it is not for the church to be a legislator for society: that is a task for politicians, for the worldly kingdom not the spiritual one. What *is* a relevant task for the church is to criticize laws and politics.

The doctrine of the two kingdoms makes it clear that God can do good things through everyone, including people who are not Christians. It is one of the tasks of the church to stress this perspective. The point is that the actor is God, not human beings.

God can use biotechnology to cure human beings and to create better conditions of life. People taking part in this work may be seen as fulfilling the mission Jesus gave the apostles to cure sick human bodies. The church has to point out that this work is a good gift from God, provided that the scientists and medical doctors respect the dignity of human beings.

But human beings also can misuse biotechnology. The consequences of that can be devastating for human beings, for animals, for the environment. Here lies the ambiguity, and this ambiguity must be recognized continually in the proclamation of the Christian message. Human beings are created good but constantly do what is wrong. Theological and Christian ethics must offer a direction to bioethics on the basis of a Christian view of life.

The limits of ethics. The church lives and works in the time between the resurrection and ascension of Christ and his return on the last day. In other words, the church is an *eschatological* entity. Yet the portrait in the New Testament of the first Christians waiting for the last day, with all its consequences for the life of Christian people, shows that they were at the same time working and planning for the future. Christian hope and daily work are not contrasts, but are intimately related to one another. The struggle of human beings must deal with welfare in this world, but it is also a task for the church to prepare human beings for eternal life.

Christian hope reaches beyond the limits of time and space, as does the struggle of human beings. The permanent struggle of human beings to cross the boundaries and break down the barriers which stand in their way is illustrated very obviously in biotechnology. But biotechnology has brought a new situation. Sometimes this is expressed in the phrase "playing God". Biotechnology gives an unprecedented power to human beings. The use of biotechnology may enable humans to change the concept of life for themselves, for animals and for the environment. Human beings manipulate the genetic code. That is why it is important to formulate moral limits on the power of human beings. It is a task for the church to proclaim that, in crossing genetic boundaries, human beings must always act in a responsible way.

The church also proclaims that in the last day God will create new heavens and a new earth. But it is important to add that the Christian hope includes not only souls but also bodies. Spirit and matter will be united. This eschatological perspective will also remind us that there is an end for the world. Political and scientific utopias are limited by the Christian doctrine of the last things. This doctrine also underscores human responsibility for the whole creation and emphasizes that creation is good. The Christian idea of the good creation and the Christian hope of a new creation protect us against nihilism and irresponsibility.

According to the Lutheran tradition, bioethics belongs to the field of law and reason. A scientific search for truth in the context of political decisions and legislation may be the starting point for a Christian discussion of bioethics. The church's task is to evaluate scientific and political reality in terms of the Christian view of creation and human beings. And so the church has to proclaim the gospel of the forgiveness of sins, the resurrection of the body and eternal life. This proclamation may be an inspiration for responsibility in time for the sake of the world.

Within the Lutheran tradition, the goal of engagement in bioethical problems may be a good development for human beings and for the whole of creation. But it should not be forgotten that there is an ultimate limit to the power of human beings: death. The Christian hope proclaims resurrection and eternal life. This belief gives inspiration to responsible life and stewardship of the whole creation: "But, in accordance with his promise, we wait for new heavens and a new earth, where righteousness is at home" (2 Peter 3:13).

From principles to applied ethics

On the basis of this view of the human being, the world, Scripture and the church, one may ask whether the Lutheran church has normative criteria which may serve as a basis for evaluating bioethical problems. What help can it offer people who are confronted with difficult ethical dilemmas in their personal life, family, occupation or as citizens and are seeking guidelines?

Bioethics involves the most fundamental Christian beliefs regarding human beings, their dignity, rights, integrity and quality of life and their health, suffering and death. In addition to the normative criteria already mentioned, the following should be emphasized:

Human dignity. As mentioned above, the constructive basis of the approach taken by the church and theology to bioethical questions must lie in the concept of creation. Human life, the body and health are gifts from God the Creator and subject to human management with personal responsibility to the Creator. In his *Small Catechism* Luther says: "I believe that God has created me and all that exists; that he has given me and still sustains my body and soul, all my limbs and senses, my reason and all the faculties of my mind..." Equally relevant to bioethics is the negative side: life, body and health are threatened as a result of death and the powers of sin among humans and in the world. The moral efforts of all human beings can thus be interpreted theologically as a protection of the benefits of creation and a struggle against transitoriness and the destructive power of sin.

Central to the Christian view of human beings is the concept of their unique value. This dignity is implied by the belief that we are created in the image of God and that we are loved by God in Jesus Christ (cf. John 3:16). The church thus operates with a theocentric and relational justification for human dignity.

In terms of content, this means that Christianity ascribes to human beings a fundamental dignity purely on the basis of their existence, not just a functional value depending on the skills they have or the tasks they fulfill. This fundamental value has universal application: it is ascribed to everyone regardless of age, sex, race or social status. Everyone is equal. It is part of practising neighbourly love to show this respect to everyone and to contribute to establishing and maintaining social institutions that express equal respect to every citizen.

But there are diverging interpretations within the Lutheran tradition of when humans attain their dignity and how absolute or inviolable it is. There are two main views on the first question. Some would hold that human dignity exists from the moment of conception. The justification for this view lies partly in the fact that relations to God, fellow human beings and their surroundings exist objectively from that time on, partly in the fact that the fertilized egg contains all potential human qualities. Others would see human dignity as something which gradually increases in relation to the development from conception to birth. This view of human life "in development", distinguishing between persons and non-persons, presupposes that full human dignity is something individuals attain over time. (These views are discussed further in the "Letter to a Medical Researcher", pp.50-63.)

The inviolability of this human dignity is an expression of the unique position of the human being in creation and its right to life. But not even Lutheran theologians define this right as absolute. At the centre of discussion here is the question of which individual and public considerations are important enough to legitimate a breach of the right to life and protection.

Human rights. Bioethics must also take into account the relevance of human rights and the degree to which a theological ethics can benefit from such an approach.

As set forth, for example, in the Universal Declaration of Human Rights of 1948, human rights are clearly related to central norms in Christian ethics (life, freedom, right to work and rest). But it is also important to see traditional human rights as anchored in the natural reason of the human being (as well as culture and history). This perspective differs from the theological one, in which the human being is always seen in his or her relation to God, and life and dignity are not rights but gifts. An ethics of fundamental or natural rights also seems to run counter to the demand of neighbourly love. The latter places an obligation on every moral agent, whereas an ethics of rights starts with entitlement of the agent.

Recent research on human rights shows that their main function is to regulate the relationship between individuals and the public in society. It is also claimed that they are open to various forms of legitimation in religious or similar contexts. Thus, the focus may shift from the foundation of the rights to their content and use. It is then theologically possible to talk about human rights *coram hominibus* and to understand rights as consistent with the overall commandment to "love your neighbour", which combines individual responsibility with a loving care for one's fellow human beings.

In a bioethical context, the fundamental right to life and freedom from physical abuse are central norms (Universal Declaration, articles 3 and 5). From a Christian perspective, both are expressed in the fifth commandment (Exodus 20:13; Matthew 19:18; Romans 13:9). Luther expressed the scope of this commandment in the following manner in his *Small Catechism*: "We shall fear and love God so that we neither injure nor do harm to [our neighbour's] body, but help and support him in all corporal need."

The scope of human rights is important in addressing individual cases in bioethics. For example, from a theological perspective, it is doubtful whether it is legitimate to speak of a fundamental right to have children and to become parents (more concerning this in the "Letter to a Childless Couple", pp.41-49).

Human integrity. In all ethics — not least in bioethics — the question of human integrity is relevant.

Integrity means that something is complete and uninjured. Used in relation to states, the concept refers to the inviolability of a country's territory. Applied to human beings, the reasoning is similar: each person has a "territory" or "life space" which must be respected by others. If the boundaries of this private sphere are crossed, the individual's personal identity is violated.

In the context of bioethics it is most relevant to point out how an individual's body is such a personal "territory" which may not be violated by others. The concept of "informed consent" prior to medical treatment can be seen as a concrete example of applying the ideal of integrity to the occupational ethics of health personnel and biomedical researchers.

Integrity can be understood as a consequence of human dignity. As such, it is appropriate to ascribe this not only to those who are born but also to the unborn, in terms of their right to be protected against physical injuries. This ethical norm does not only apply to pregnant women using drugs or other substances injurious to human foetuses. It could also be applied when assessing the problems of research on foetuses and the use of foetal tissue. In recent years there has been discussion of whether the norm of integrity applies not only to human body parts and organs but also to human genes. Scientific advances are making this discussion more and more crucial, but no satisfactory consensus has yet been reached.

Quality of life. The concept "quality of life" has been used in modern bioethics, sometimes descriptively to refer to the health of a person, sometimes normatively to prescribe a course of action. But it has proved difficult to give the concept a sufficiently precise content for it to serve as a fruitful criterion for ethical reflection.

When used as an ethical norm, "quality of life" has usually been given a teleological or consequentialist ethical interpretation: in other words, the question of duties with respect to human life and the body must also take into consideration people's capabilities and practice of them. The qualities most often mentioned are reason, happiness and intelligence.

The concept of quality of life seems to include two components. On the one hand, there are some "objective" requirements which must be met, such as bodily functions, fulfillment of basic needs, opportunities and so on. On the other hand, quality of life is a question of how the individual experiences his or her own life. Is he or she happy? Does he or she "feel good" about life? In the biomedical sphere the concept of quality of life plays a role in the discussion about what health is, what to do when treatment becomes futile and how to distribute scarce resources in health care. In all these contexts efforts have been made to find measures for quality of life.

The ambiguities in the concept of quality of life can be dangerous. If we try to find an objective measure of it, we will inevitably come to judge that some individuals have a lower quality of life than others; and then we run the risk of saying that a person with a certain low quality of life is not as important as others. Thus thinking along the lines of quality of life can lead to violating the basic idea of equal human dignity.

This danger should not prevent us from recognizing that there is an important moral idea behind this notion: the idea of the "good life". From the standpoint of Christian neighbourly love, the good is in the first instance the good I am obliged to do to the other. In order to show neighbourly love, we always have to find the middle way between merely being an instrument for fulfilling the desires of the other and practising tutelage as though we know best what is good for others. A similar balance must be expected from society: it should secure every citizen the minimum of goods necessary to lead a decent life, but under no circumstances does it have the right to say that some people are not worth treatment or regard because their quality of life is too low.

Health, suffering and death. Theologically, health is a gift from the Creator and illness is a consequence of the transitoriness of human beings and the destructive effect of the fall on the entire creation. These destructive consequences form a continual calling to engagement for the benefit of fellow beings. Viewed as a God-created value and in the light of the protection of the body mandated by the fifth commandment, the concern for health underlines the ethical responsibility all persons have for their own and others' physical, mental and social capability.

The questions of quality of life and health also give rise to another issue: should freedom from suffering not be a central value in the work of bioethics? Without a doubt the concept of suffering is generally relevant in such bioethical areas as IVF, abortion, organ transplants, suicide, euthanasia and others.

From the theological perspective of divine creation, efforts to eliminate or reduce physical, psychological and other suffering are a legitimate expression of our struggle against imperfection and evil. For ethical reflection, it is particularly important to examine any possible conflicts between the value of freedom from suffering and life itself. It must be maintained that a life without suffering is not an absolute ethical ideal. Such a life has priority second to the confirmation of the biological existence. Alleviation of pain is still a central issue, ethically considered. In the case of unavoidable suffering, the task may be to maintain inter-human relations as a burden-carrying fellowship.

Finally, a Lutheran bioethics must include an overall biblically founded perspective on death. On the one hand, death is a consequence of the source of human beings in the "dust of the ground" (Genesis 2:7; cf. Psalm 104:29). Understood this way, biological death is something natural. On the other hand, it is also a punishment for sin (Genesis 2:17, 3:1ff.; Psalms 90:3, 7-9; Romans 5:12ff.; 1 Corinthians 15:21f.). Understood in this manner, death is an enemy.

Applied to concrete bioethical problems, this means that in the face of a situation in which a person is in the process of enduring a long and painful death, it is theologically legitimate to view death as a "prescript" for all creation and a gift offering liberation from human pain. Death must at the same time also be seen as a judgment over humanity collectively, sometimes resulting in a difficult shortening of a person's life. Questions involving euthanasia can serve to illustrate that both aspects are often relevant in individual cases of death.

Part Two

Community and Bioethics

Eight Letters

3. *Genetic Counselling and Prenatal Diagnosis*

An Exchange between a Medical Doctor and a Theologian

KEES VAN KOOTEN NIEKERK
and PER SUNDSTRÖM

Dear Pastor Smith,

I am writing to you because I think it might be useful for me to get some advice before giving advice on a situation that has arisen in my medical practice. This has to do with genetic counselling.

Recently I was contacted for advice by a married couple with two children who are thinking of having another baby. This sounds innocent enough, but it isn't, since the second of their two children, a three-year-old boy, suffers from cystic fibrosis (CF). This is a genetic disease. It can be predicted that it will be inherited, on average, by 25 percent of the children of parents who are both healthy so-called carriers of a recessive gene for the disease on one of their chromosomes. If one gene for the disease from the mother and one from the father happen to meet in the offspring, the result will be CF; and statistically speaking this will happen to one in four children of carrier-parents. Since one child of this couple has the disease, we know that these parents are carriers, which means a 25 percent chance that another pregnancy will result in a diseased child.

Clinically speaking, CF is a disease that affects the lungs, the pancreas and often several other organs. Secretions of various substances are distorted, and thick mucus accumulates in the lungs and the pancreas. The tissues of the affected organs degenerate, form cysts and eventually become fibrous (hence the name CF). Breathing gradually becomes more difficult, and the lungs, in which mucus accumulates, become fertile soil for repeated infections. This is often the first sign of the disease already in the infant or small child. Symptoms of malabsorption and malnutrition due to pancreatic insufficiency will also usually show up early.

There is no treatment that cures the basic defect. Available treatment includes antibiotics against the lung infections, enzymes to substitute for the insufficient pancreas and physical therapy to get rid of the viscous mucus in the lungs. Thanks to intensive therapeutic interventions from an early age, CF patients often survive until early adulthood. But eventually the disease is fatal. Perhaps I should add that CF is a fairly common disease in most countries in Europe and America; about one child in two thousand is affected.

In cases like that of the couple seeking my advice, one may be quite sure the parents do want to have another child. They are beginning to know what it is like to live with a child suffering from CF — a tough life for them as well as for the child. They are informed about their status as carriers of the gene for the disease, and they understand the pattern of inheritance. They would not take another pregnancy lightly. Yet I was careful to confirm that they really wish to have another child. They do.

I went on to inform them about the current state of prenatal diagnosis regarding CF. Between the ninth and eleventh weeks of pregnancy a chorionic villus sampling is performed: a small sample of the chorionic villi (finger-like projections) of the placenta is removed by inserting a thin needle through the mother's abdominal wall or via a catheter through the vagina into the uterus. When the genetic material (DNA) of these cells is analyzed, it can be ascertained with a high degree of accuracy whether or not the foetus has inherited the gene from both parents and thus whether it will acquire the disease. If it turns out that the foetus will develop CF, abortion is an option, since the test result is available so early in pregnancy.

Having said that much, I thought I had done what I could and should in order to help and support this couple. But already the same evening I began to have second thoughts. Had I been too quick to suggest prenatal diagnosis and then to propose abortion as an option that is always open to any pregnant woman? Was I prejudiced? Had I listened to them carefully enough? Had I perhaps taken the moral issues of prenatal diagnosis and abortion too lightly?

I would like to know how you look on a case like this one as someone who has reflected on these issues from a moral and religious point of view. Of course, I will have to handle the case myself; I am not expecting you to say: "Do this, don't do that." But I do think you will have something to say that might help me see things more clearly.

Yours sincerely,
George Brown, M.D.

Dear Dr Brown,

Thank you for your letter. I am honoured by the confidence you demonstrate by asking my advice.

Let me begin by saying that, as far as I can tell from your story, no serious objection can be made to what you have done and said in this case. On the contrary, you seem to have handled it carefully and sensibly — professionally, in the best sense of the word. Yet you have had some second thoughts; and it is never wise to try to silence second thoughts before considering them carefully. In that process you may find some of my comments helpful. But remember: I am an outsider, and it is precisely as an outsider that I may help you. You are the one to make up your mind in this case. There is no substitute for that.

Correct, unbiased medical information is of course essential in a case like this. Ignorance in a physician is a basic fault, but so is the failure to communicate the knowledge one has. While this is usually taken for granted in medical ethics, I think it is worth pointing out, given how complicated and powerful modern medicine is.

Equally essential in a case like this is to let the couple come out with their feelings, thoughts and questions. This requires attentiveness on the physician's part and may take time; but what the couple have to say is no less important than the medical information. They ought to feel they are taking part in a decision-making process, not waiting to hear the physician tell them what they are supposed to do. This is important not least from a moral point of view: there are choices to be made, and the medical information provided by the physician does not decide the case.

The physician should also make it clear that there may be three decisions for the couple to make. First, should we have another child? Second, should we accept prenatal diagnosis? Third, should we abort a foetus that will later develop CF? The first question ought to be answered first; and without a clear "yes" it is doubtful whether one ought to proceed to the second. Furthermore, if prenatal diagnosis has been performed and has shown that the child will acquire CF, it should not be forgotten that there is still one question to be asked, namely the one about abortion. That is a new decision; it has not been decided by saying "yes" to prenatal diagnosis. Here the physician must be careful not to insinuate that a CF diagnosis makes abortion the "natural" solution.

Generally speaking, abortion would almost always be questionable. It terminates the life of a human being *in spe*. Every human being is created in the image of God and loved by God; and the dignity of a human being surpasses that of any other creature. This means that from a Christian point of view, abortion can only be a last resort, when the mental or physical health of the mother is seriously threatened by the pregnancy, or when it can be predicted that the child, if it were born, would have a short life of severe suffering. A child, if allowed to be born, may also under certain conditions become a serious threat to the life and community of a family (I shall come back to this point shortly). These predictions are difficult to make, especially for an outsider like myself. You and the parents are in a better position to make them.

Of course one has to take into account that there is already a child suffering from CF in this family. As you wrote in your letter, their everyday life is already difficult, and it would probably grow tougher if there were another child with CF in the family. It would be insensitive not to understand that the parents may wish to have a prenatal diagnosis performed, and that they may think of abortion as a way out if the foetus should turn out to have inherited the disease. They must ask themselves if they would have the strength to take care of two children suffering from CF. If not, the whole family could be put into jeopardy. In that case an abortion might be the lesser of two evils. But then they should also ask themselves anew whether it would be better to refrain from having another child in the first place.

The physician should not try to push them in either direction. It is their decision, supported one may hope by family and friends. It is easy to be morally radical when you do not have to bear the consequences. Moral concern for the welfare of the foetus can degenerate into self-righteousness and a disregard for anxious and ambivalent parents. This point is also reinforced by our religious tradition: love is the ultimate moral criterion, but love is incompatible with a self-righteous attitude.

These are my reflections after reading your letter. As you yourself have said, the response is yours; and I feel confident you will make the best of it. I suppose — and hope — that you will meet with this couple again, after they have had some time to think it over.

With best wishes for your work,

Yours sincerely,
David Smith, D.D.

4. *In Vitro Fertilization*

A Letter to a Childless Couple

BJÖRN BJÖRNSSON and LENA KJEMS

Dear Rachel and Jacob,

I was deeply moved by your letter, with its heart-breaking description of the pain you experience in not being able to have a child of your own; and I can well understand how recent developments in reproductive technologies have brought renewed hope into your lives. You ask if there is any reason whatsoever not to join a fertility programme. While your question seemed somewhat rhetorical, I also sensed a deep concern on your part to make the right choice.

I want to emphasize at the beginning the importance of making certain that our choices are *informed*. With all the dramatic technological developments in our day, we are often not all that impressed when we hear about yet another "scientific breakthrough". However, there are occasions which we sense are of outstanding significance, truly epoch-making in fundamentally affecting our worldview. One such event was the first man on the moon, another the first test-tube baby. If walking on the moon is seen as a symbol of the gigantic human outreach into the universe, the making of the first child *in vitro* heralded the entry into the deep mystery of the beginning of human life. How these two developments affect us personally is worlds apart. The moon is still just as much "out of reach" for most of us as it always has been; whereas a "test-tube baby" is now the much-desired and beloved child of many formerly distressed childless couples who have become happy parents.

What makes reproductive technology different from most other technological advances is the extraordinary importance it may have for our most cherished and personal concerns. For couples who have had to face the fact that their sexual union will not bring forth a child of their own, there are now technical means available to overcome childlessness, which many have experienced as a personal tragedy. My concern in this letter is to share with you some of the ideas and questions that seem to me to arise when Christian faith and ethics are brought to bear on the radical new situation childless couples now face. Christian communities are obliged to take an active part in the public debate on the many complicated moral issues that come in the wake of new developments in medicine and the life sciences.

Reproductive technology is of particular concern to the churches since the institution of marriage and the family, which has always been central in the Christian message, is greatly affected by the good, but also the possible evil, of this technology. On the positive side, it is safe to assume that the church will universally welcome efforts aimed at finding a solution to infertility. Children are seen as a gift of God, a blessing on marriage, one of the basic goods of family life. But this may be as far as the churches are able to speak with one voice when evaluating what speaks for and against the most recent developments in reproductive technology. Underlying the reasons for the different views the churches will take are theological differences on important issues, such as the sanctity of marriage, family life and alternative forms of family organization, procreation and artificial means of contraception and reproduction, just to mention a few. Besides that, one may expect that committed church people will share with the general public much the same concerns which mark the bioethical debate in general.

Reproductive technology can be defined as the biotechnological reconstruction of human procreation. The basic procedure here is *in vitro* fertilization (IVF), which is fertilization outside the female body. Breakthroughs in the techniques for doing this seem indeed to have brought miracles into the life of many infertile couples. Still, I want to try in this letter to point to some of the profound moral questions which the practice of reproductive technology raises, both for individual couples and for society as a whole. It is indeed the significance of life itself that these new technologies may come to shape and alter.

From my perspective as a Lutheran, a starting-point for ethics could be the recognition of a certain latitude in moral questions. Applied to this question, that means that there is no command from above about which reproductive choices we shall make. So I see my task in this letter as a more modest one: describing some moral issues involved in reproductive technology so as to help you as a childless couple to make a morally responsible choice of your own. Framing the relevant moral questions may prove just as helpful as providing the answers. However, at least two concepts in the Christian faith mark out a framework within which a tentative evaluation of IVF can be made.

1. *The gospel takes a preferential option for the poor and vulnerable*. This may shed some light on the question of whom to care about within a biotechnological context. Identifying and protecting the vulnerable is a significant concern of the moral enterprise within a Lutheran context. IVF procedures often involve third parties or they affect the persons involved in a disproportionate way. Consequently, reproductive technology can be assessed on the basis of if and how justice is served, interpersonally and globally.

2. *Human beings are never to be used only as a means; human value is not instrumental but intrinsic*. We are not valuable because of our reproductive capacities, but we have value as loved by God; and we transmit this love in working for the well-being of our neighbour. A biologically related child is not the only proper object for our human desire to love and to be loved. The transformation of the family in the teachings of Jesus illustrates this point. This of course does not mean that the desire for biological offspring is morally suspect. The family has been highly regarded within the Lutheran tradition, carrying on the Old Testament notion of the family as a sign of God's blessing. Luther himself used the imagery of parental authority to illustrate God's authority. Life as a gift is a fundamental notion cherished in the Christian tradition, meaning that biological offspring can be viewed as a very concrete way of passing on this gift.

In the following, I shall try to evaluate reproductive technologies in the light of these concerns. I will distinguish among three ways of employing the techniques of *in vitro* fertilization: the standard case of IVF, IVF by donor and IVF and genetic engineering. I will give more emphasis to the first two, since the real breakthrough in gene-therapy still belongs to the future.

The standard case of IVF

The most straightforward type of IVF involves a married couple — a man and a woman — who undergo the procedure without involving others. We read about something of the grief and sadness involuntary infertility causes in biblical stories (for example, that of Rachel in Genesis 30). Ethics from a Lutheran perspective acknowledges that tremendous pain, and the traditional Lutheran appreciation of family may help explain why many Lutheran communities have accepted IVF as a way of enabling otherwise infertile couples to have children. However, this acceptance has been provisional, since IVF poses serious problems in relation to at least three issues: abortion, gender justice and global justice.

Objections have been made in the first place to the disposal and waste of fertilized eggs and embryos during the process of fertilization and gestation. Even if embryo loss does not constitute abortion in the strict sense of the term, some have questioned the disregard of human material which is implied in these procedures. To say that reproductive technologies are life-creating procedures is thus only part of the truth. The day may come when the techniques of IVF will be perfected so that no genetic material has to be discarded; and this will no doubt take away some of the reservations Christians have expressed about it. However, there is still the question of vocabulary to be dealt with. Such scientific designations as “embryo” and “genetic material” veil the fact that we are referring to potential human beings, who must be treated in a dignified way. Reproductive technology has brought about a situation where human embryos can exist outside any type of human relationship.

Second, the desire for a child of one’s own puts the infertile woman in a vulnerable position. It is she who has to undergo invasive medical treatment with no guarantee of success. Nothing is yet known about the long-term effects on a woman of heavy hormonal treatment and egg-retrieval. Women are more socially stigmatized than men for infertility, since bearing children has been seen culturally as the essence of femininity.

Furthermore, external fertilization provides the medical community with information that may make it the experts of the procreation process at the expense of women’s experience. Reproductive medicine has become a prestigious area of research that depends upon women's bodies; and conflicts of interests may arise when treatment and research are intermingled. More broadly, when procreation is set within reproductive technology, does the female loss of control affect the bonding process between woman and child? Does the "medicalization" of fertilization, pregnancy and birth alter the significance of life?

Moreover, although unwanted childlessness may be a devastating experience, infertility is not a disease. It is not easy to defend the practice of women undergoing invasive bodily procedures because of their husbands' infertility. It is worth asking why more and more people become infertile. In recent years growing attention has been paid to environmental factors. Much more funding is needed for research aimed at elucidating easily preventable causes for infertility.

In the third place, IVF is expensive. That means few couples — and most of them are in the Western world — can afford it. So, paradoxically, while some are spending great amounts of money to obtain biological offspring, thousands of children around the world are dying from starvation every day. Seen globally, reproductive technology, broadly understood as any technique related to human procreation, may reinforce asymmetrical power relations. Reproductive technologies may be used in the so-called third world in order to practise population control. Moreover, the idea of female inferiority in certain cultures is being reinforced by technology in the form of amniocentesis. This procedure makes it possible to detect the sex of the foetus, which can then be aborted if it is a girl. When these techniques become more advanced and it becomes possible to engineer sex before fertilization occurs, it will be even easier to act on such old prejudices.

The issue of adoption needs to be dealt with in the context of reproductive technology. To what extent does this present a suitable alternative to IVF? Adoption would seem to be one way of realizing the human potential for giving and receiving love, which ought not to be confined to biological relations. In any case it is objectionable that in some countries a couple signing up for IVF within the public health system must take their name off official adoption lists. And while persons are allowed into a fertility programme with almost no questions asked, adoption procedures are extremely difficult.

The idea that biological offspring is a human right is increasingly heard in the Western public debate. Certainly the liberal tradition at least has acknowledged the right to procreation without interference from outside, but there has never been a right to biological offspring at any cost. With all the new options available through IVF, it is first of all the rights *of* the child that we must consider, rather than any presumed "right *to* a child". A child is a gift, never to be considered as a piece of property. Acceptance of the child as a gift of God is an expression of the fundamental human birthright as being created in the image of God, male and female. As we acknowledge the gift of life to us, our "birthright", we commit ourselves to live up to our calling by respecting and furthering the same right in the lives of others. This is supremely the case when we as parents are entrusted with the gift of a child.

This important theological context suggests the need for a pronounced child-centred approach to the moral dilemmas raised by reproductive technology. A key concept here is the notion of responsible parenthood. Moral responsibility will then unfold as an emphasis on parental obligations rather than parental rights. Responsible parenthood is intimately linked with the Lutheran teaching of vocation. Luther believed that every station in life carries the calling to serve the neighbour. Marriage and the family were primarily important for him as a community of love and neighbourly service, a calling to be honoured not least in the fulfilment of parental duties. Today, when these truths need to be presented in a radically different context, I suggest that the concept of responsible parenthood will serve this end quite well. One very relevant element of the different social and cultural context to be taken account of is the present-day plurality of systems of family organization. The emphasis on responsible parenthood as a moral criterion means that all forms of family living are set under its scrutiny: heterosexual unions of various types, the single-parent family and homosexual partnerships.

Recognition of responsible parenthood as a guiding principle can be of great help to us not only as a moral community but also as concerned individuals. It may play an important part in deciding on the limits beyond which the application of reproductive technology cannot be morally justified. It can also serve as a guideline for childless couples in making a moral choice of their own in their concrete circumstances. I said earlier that there is no command from above in this area. That makes it all the more important that we consider carefully and well how reproductive choices shall be made. It is with this in mind that I emphasize responsible parenthood as a moral guideline. It involves no infringement on individual moral responsibility, but recognizes at the same time that there is no virtue in leaving those burdened with a heavy moral responsibility altogether unassisted.

IVF by donor

If a couple is unable to provide the genetic material necessary for fertilization, they may obtain ova or semen from donors. With today's advanced techniques both ova and semen may come from donors, so that neither of the parents-to-be provides any genetic material. The moral questions increase with each additional person involved, particularly the question of who are the vulnerable parties in IVF by donor. One is the donor, another the child to be. It is not unlikely that it is the less privileged who will pay the price — as donors of all types. One way of avoiding this form of exploitation has been to utilize surplus eggs from women enrolled in fertility programmes. But with the improvement of fertilization techniques surplus eggs become fewer and fewer. It is important to keep in mind that the marketplace is not the proper sphere for the reproduction of human life and the commercialization of procreation must be questioned: any biotechnological procedure that involves the buying and selling of reproductive services must be regarded with suspicion.

Biotechnological motherhood can be split among three persons: the woman who provides the ova, the woman who bears and gives birth to the child and the woman who brings up the child. In certain cases it will require the wisdom of Solomon to settle the issue of who is the mother. IVF by donor complicates greatly the application of the crucial principle of our maxim of "responsible parenthood": that it is our duty always to give precedence to the rights of the child. This is implicit in the concept of parenthood, especially seen in the context of a preferential option for the poor and vulnerable. Perhaps the most basic right of a child is to be able to identify with its parents, to know them and, what is even more important, to be known by them and loved by them. It is sad but true that children have often been deprived of this right by their biological parents, but of course that in no way justifies that a very important part of this right now be systematically taken away from them.

How does a child identify with three "mothers", as in the example above (and much more complex cases of confused identities could be cited)? The involvement of a donor in the process of procreation established a threat to children's rights from the earliest days of reproductive technology in the form of artificial insemination by donor (AID). Now with IVF, the questionable effects of donation on the well-being of children multiply as ever-new combinations are offered by the advancing technology. With this in mind, and in respect of the command of responsible parenthood, it is my conviction that IVF should be reserved for couples for whom no donation is needed.

IVF and genetic engineering

The use of IVF in connection with prenatal diagnostics and other kinds of genetic engineering raises profound moral questions. Screening techniques to detect abnormalities in the fertilized egg seem to render therapeutic abortion superfluous. Many will regard this as a major moral achievement, as it surely will be. Detection of serious genetic disorders at an early stage will avoid the trauma of having a late abortion. In the longer run, refinement of techniques of gene therapy will make it possible to perform foetal surgery and avoid abortion altogether.

Within this context of new genetic possibilities, a high degree of responsibility will be called for, since it may become possible not only to have a child but to a certain degree to decide what kind of child is wanted. I have already mentioned the issue of sex-selection without any therapeutic reason, but the possibilities in this area seem endless. Patterns of exclusion are presumably at work in the practice of new reproductive technologies. The almost exclusive focus on the childless couple and their desire for biological offspring may reduce the role of other significant actors to a purely instrumental one: egg- or sperm-donor, surrogate mother.

I believe there is a morally significant difference between the standard case of IVF — the couple with no need to involve others — and IVF by donor or IVF in connection with genetic engineering. Provided that the woman is fully aware of the various risks to herself and that the couple has a stable and loving relationship, the mere artificiality of the procedure does not justify a general ban on IVF. IVF involving donation is morally more ambiguous, since consideration must be shown for both the donor and the child-to-be. It is difficult at this stage to predict the development of genetic engineering within the area of reproduction. Time will tell whether it will be possible to maintain a sharp distinction between different types of IVF.

Dear friends, I wish you the very best in the future, and I hope this letter may help you in making the right decision and, not least, that it will come true.

Best regards,
Your friend, Martin

5. *Fertilized Eggs and Pre-Implantation Diagnosis*

A Letter to a Medical Researcher

LARS ØSTNOR and ANNE-MARIE THUNBERG

Dear Hera,

A heartfelt thank you for your interesting and engaging letter. In an instructive way you have managed to inform us about your daily research work at the hospital. Now you would like to know what we as representatives of the Lutheran church in your country think about the burning ethical challenges you are confronted with. The first has to do with how we are to understand a fertilized egg — its moral value and its eventual right to protection from individuals and society. Second, you ask about our position of principle regarding the legitimacy and boundaries of research from an ethical point of view. Maybe you have raised this question out of a sense that you as a researcher are not receiving sufficient support from theological or church quarters concerning the effort you and others are making to gain new and useful insight in the field of human reproduction. Finally, you would like to hear what theology might contribute to ethical norms and values that might provide constructive ethical guidelines for responsible work in your field.

All three questions focus on the most debated and discussed areas of concern in today's bioethics. In the hope that we might come to a fruitful interdisciplinary exchange of opinion, we would like in this letter to offer our own evaluation of the problems facing all of us.

All three areas of concern you mention are linked to our dealings with fertilized eggs in the form of research and diagnosis in the earliest phase of human life. But on the basis of your letter as well as the reading we have done, it seems to us that there are several parts of a larger field of problems which need to be dealt with separately.

First of all the concept "fertilized eggs" deserves a closer explanation. As you know even better than we do, a large variety of expressions are used in describing the development of a human life from fertilization to birth. When one speaks of a fertilized egg, it usually refers to the phase of development which takes place during the first 14 days. In medical literature we have read, the terms "blastem", "zygote" and "pre-embryo" are also used for this. The term "embryo" is used for the following period, which lasts up to the eighth week; from then on one uses the term "foetus". In many articles and much of the public debate, embryo seems the most common terminology. Here we prefer to speak of fertilized eggs, just to underscore that our topic is the new human life in the first weeks of its existence.

In our view the language is not decisive unless with the help of different descriptions one tries to draw a line of principle, thereby distinguishing the different phases from one another. Such a separation, which could eventually have important practical consequences with regard to our dealings with human life, is hardly relevant. Biological development from fertilization to birth is according to today's knowledge a continuous process which proceeds without any qualitative leaps that would make it possible to identify any evident periods.

Second, because research on fertilized eggs is a relatively new phenomenon, there is not much of an ethical tradition to draw upon. It is especially through *in vitro* fertilization (IVF) that these questions have come to the fore. The process of "tubular fertilization" leaves some redundant fertilized eggs, since not all of them are put in the woman's womb. Since you are working in a ward where such treatment is given, we suppose that the fertilized eggs to which you have access are the so-called "spare eggs" remaining after the IVF-treatment of infertile couples. As far as we know, one can work with these eggs outside the mother's body for up to one week before they begin to be destroyed.

In reflecting on our ethical responsibility towards such eggs, it might be fruitful to distinguish between research of a more clinical character on eggs which are to be brought back to the woman and cases in which eggs are used solely for research purposes. In the former case the researcher might change the temperature and the consistency of the medium in which the fertilized egg is kept before implantation in order to ensure the best possible development for the egg. This does not cause any change in the genetic material or destroy the egg. In the latter case we are talking about fertilized eggs which are not being implanted and which are exposed to treatment of which one does not know the consequences. The aim is increased knowledge, and the consequence is that the eggs are destroyed. We understand from your letter that it is this latter case — research which can be said to consume fertilized eggs in the process — about which you are especially eager to challenge us as church representatives.

But even here we may be dealing with varied problems. Researchers may have different motives for seeking knowledge from the study of fertilized eggs before they are destroyed. It may be for the purpose of improving the technique used for IVF: it may be to gain more insight into the first phases of human life (embryology); it may be to find ways of diagnosing possible genetic diseases before the egg is implanted in the womb (pre-implantation diagnosis). We shall deal with these situations one-by-one.

Fertilized eggs: their ethical status

Any approach to the question of what is "right" or "good" in research on fertilized eggs should begin by asking what value we should assign to a fertilized human egg. You probably know that innumerable answers have been given to this question from the perspectives of natural science, philosophy, theology and other disciplines. Within the scope of this letter, we have to deal with these rather summarily.

From the perspective of natural sciences like biology and medicine, it has been argued that the physical process from fertilization to birth justifies according human beings an increasing value that is related to and rooted in this development. From this one can deduce that a human being's value starts at zero, is low for a zygote and reaches its full measure at birth. By graduating the value in this way, one can agree that it is ethically legitimate to deal with a fertilized egg in a way no one would defend if it were a fully developed foetus.

Philosophers have proposed various ways of distinguishing between the human being as a biological entity and as a person. It is common in such conceptions to hold that not every individual belonging to the species *homo sapiens* meets the qualifications to be considered a person. A "person" is one who possesses certain defined characteristics related to different capacities. The qualities or standards used may vary somewhat from one philosopher to another, but generally speaking they include reason, consciousness, the ability to communicate and the like. Only human beings with these capacities are ascribed their full value and the right to life and protection. How one is to think of human organisms which are not (as yet) persons varies. Usually their value is counted as partial and related to the degree of development. Fertilized eggs which are not implanted, as a consequence, have minimal value or none at all, though some philosophers attach value to such eggs on the ground that they have the potential to develop to human beings of full worth.

On the theological scene there is a certain difference between, for example, the Roman Catholic and the Lutheran positions. The official teaching of the Catholic magisterium upholds the principle that human beings from conception onwards are to be respected as persons and that it is a moral obligation to protect human life in its entirety. Among Lutheran theologians different tendencies have been apparent. There are those who give their argumentation on bioethical questions a specifically Christian basis, pointing to the fact that the human being is created by God and has infinite value. Others choose to put forward their arguments on a more common basis by ascribing human dignity either to personality or to the fact that each individual as a part of humankind is to be understood collectively. The important difference between these two lines of thinking is illustrated by the question of research on fertilized eggs and embryos which will not be implanted. The former group of theologians are negative about this kind of research, referring to a full, non-graded worth of human being starting from the time of conception. The latter operate with another understanding of the dignity of humankind: it is graded and subject to change depending on the biological level of development. In this case it is permissible under certain conditions to conduct research on eggs and embryos. Finally, some theologians try to combine these two lines of thought: the concept that the human being is created by God according to his image is added to the concept of biological development. This leads to the idea of a human being's value as graded. In this attempt at a synthesis, it is not always clear at which point one begins to ascribe full worth to the human being.

Some of what you wrote in your letter suggests to us that your personal sympathies run in the direction of the natural scientific (and perhaps philosophical) considerations referred to. You might like to know where we would place ourselves on the spectrum of theological positions, and how we would argue for our own position. In fact, the two of us have partly common and partly different views on this point.

To begin with what we have in common, both of us are critical of natural scientific positions which operate with a narrow evolutionary perspective, using only knowledge from biology without taking account of important ethical aspects. Likewise, we are sceptical about philosophical arguments that tend to restrict the understanding of personhood in terms of human beings, meeting certain qualitative standards. The idea that a human being is not a person from conception on, but becomes one as certain characteristics appear, is rooted in Greek tradition. Aristotle held that at a certain point in a pregnancy the foetus was bestowed with a soul (boys earlier than girls!); and Thomas Aquinas carried this idea further in Catholic theology. However, since the Enlightenment, philosophy has been influenced by the position of Immanuel Kant that the human being is a person only by virtue of his or her reason. Against this it can be argued that the concept of the human being here is ahistorical and abstract in relation to what is normally considered a "human being". The standard being used is nothing else than that of a grown up, conscious and thinking human being. Looking at the vast diversity within humanity, one can ask if we have in common any other feature than originating from a woman's egg cell and a man's seed cell. This leads us to the conclusion that it is conception which is constitutive for what is to be a human being.

To the idea that a fertilized egg or embryo has a potential for becoming a human being, one can object that such language expresses the idea of the possibilities belonging to such a life but does not include the already existing, active evolution of life taking place.

One must ask whether philosophical distinctions between biological existence and characteristics which can be said to be constitutive for personhood mix together person and subject, understood as the active self-consciousness. Thus, we are not convinced by the arguments of those who try to establish a gulf between living as a part of the species *homo sapiens* on the one hand and having a moral status as a human being of full worth on the other.

However, on the question of research on fertilized eggs our ways diverge in part, in terms of both argumentation and in conclusion. Let us try to clarify this.

Anne-Marie starts from the presupposition that the value of the human being is unconditionally valid as a principle for action. This value is due to everyone regardless of specific qualities or life conditions and throughout the whole life-cycle. Since it is not evident from biological premises at which moment in the life process the human being becomes a person, ethical reflection must stipulate that the very coming into existence is decisive. Since conception is the common point of departure for the development of all human beings, and since human value is due to the human being through the whole of life, human value should be anchored in conception.

From the basic principle that every human being possesses and should be granted human value the correlative norm follows that every human being has an inalienable right to live. This unconditioned claim for human value does not imply that there are no circumstances under which human life may be sacrificed. But when the value which an individual life must yield to is so high that one is motivated and prepared in a kind of ethical balancing act to pay the high price of a human life, one is also obliged to admit that human life is being violated, not merely reduced. To infringe upon the life of a human being always means a violation of its human value. But the principle of an unconditioned human value has to be confronted with the realities of a conditioned life-value.

This general reasoning leads to the conclusion that the principle of human value is an unconditional and indispensable instrument in ethical reflection. But it does not define what must be done when a conflict of aim or clash of values appears. In that situation it is still possible that one life must yield to another. One must draw up a balance of the values at stake, for which the principle of proportionality should be decisive: that is, what price (for example, the fertilized egg) should be paid by the value (for example, a more secure foetus development) which should be favoured? To put it another way, human value is a necessary but not sufficient precondition for moral decisions.

Lars agrees with Anne-Marie in her concern for maintaining the unique value of human beings and everyone's right to live. But he believes it is important to formulate a specific theological basis for this normative element. This he finds in the belief in creation. Human life is not only a product of decisions made by human beings but is also rooted in God's will and power to create. Each individual receives life from the Creator as a gift mediated through his or her parents. As the crown of creation, human beings have been given a unique status (theologically expressed in the phrase "created in the image of God"). We have God as Father and are fellow human beings and stewards of creation. This particular stance in relation to God, other human beings and nature provides the basis for our uniqueness. Because this value rests on its relation to God, it does not depend on characteristics, activity or work. Thus the value of the human being cannot be graduated according to a phase in life.

This does not mean that the different biological stages of development are of no interest for theology. To be a human being is always to change one's biological characteristics: growing, ageing and so on. But such phases do not warrant holding that there are qualitative leaps which legitimate degrees of human dignity. From conception onwards God is the creator of the human being, who receives his or her God-given life. Therefore, a fertilized egg has human dignity and as a consequence a right to life and protection and to maintain its possibility to develop as a human being.

This point of view does not ignore the possibility of respect for a fertilized egg being in conflict with other ethical concerns. But a consequence of it is that within such a conflict there can hardly be any relevant ethical interest vital enough to be given priority over the right to life of a fertilized egg or embryo.

Research and ethics

Your second question concerns how we are to view this kind of research. Perhaps it will be helpful to begin with some remarks about the point of view of theologians and the church regarding research in general and your kind of research in particular.

1. Theology and the church tend to have a positive evaluation of the different kinds of research. This view is rooted in the conviction that research to discover new insights into humankind and the world

around us responds to the task given to human beings to be stewards of God's creation (Genesis 1:26-28). It follows that work like this can be seen as willed by God. Research can be understood as a development of humanity's God-given resources to "put the earth under his feet" for the benefit of both nature and persons.

2. Research in itself is sometimes viewed as a kind of activity that is ethically neutral. Ethical guidelines are considered to be relevant only at that point in the process when the results of the research are being used for some kind of purpose.

This approach is far too simplistic, as is evident in the case of biomedical research. In the research that you and others are doing, the human being is not only the subject of research but also its object and aim. This requires us to ask questions of a more fundamental character: what is permissible to do with a human life during different phases of its development? what actually constitutes a human being as a human being? what consequences for human life can be tolerated? This places us squarely in the middle of a debate about the connection between anthropology and ethics. Another reason that research cannot escape ethics is that it is part of the structure and function of our societies. Research demands vast resources of personnel and economy; it provides the premises for policy decisions; it makes health care possible; it leads to the development of new technology. All of this raises questions about the means and aims of society, in other words, questions that also have ethical aspects.

Like all research, biomedical research is not insulated from ethics. It must be subject to critical scrutiny on ethical premises. Different forms of research and scientific programmes must be submitted to evaluation rooted in central ethical norms and values to determine whether they are in accord with them. There is no complete freedom of research allowing researchers simply to overlook their own ethical responsibility.

3. For persons like you who belong to a scientific milieu, a subculture develops with certain ideals and values — as it does with other groups and professions. While we do not know your situation from the inside, we know that such groups are often influenced by such factors as a dependency on new trends or what might be "in" within this particular field, a desire to advance by means of new scientific results, a sense of serving a higher imperative and being

compelled to find new methods and better technology, a general appetite for more knowledge, a tendency to select research projects primarily according to the availability for financial support and the like.

Faced with these and other internal and external demands, it is very important for a researcher like you to keep a distance and look at the situation self-critically. For doing this it helps to ask what are the main purposes of the whole range of activities being undertaken. It will probably be useful to maintain good contacts with society at large through information about one's own work and participation in the public debate about the difficult choices to be made. Of course, it should be a high priority for researchers to develop their own competence within research ethics. Finally it is necessary to look at the connection between the research and the use of it.

On this last point, a relevant question is that of how to deal with results from research undertaken on a basis that we find ethically deplorable. Can correct use justify unethical research? Our general opinion is that valuable and useful results are not enough to legitimate research that might be labelled unethical on, for instance, fertilized eggs. The research project itself must stand on its own feet. On the other hand, if research is labelled unethical, this does not prevent us from using the results when they actually exist, and might prove to serve a purpose. But a precondition of a more detailed reflection in this area is that we keep in mind whether the research has been completed or is still in progress. Moreover, one must balance the degree of fault in the research with the degree of purpose in the eventual use.

4. As you certainly know, several ethical guidelines have been worked out which are relevant to research in your field. Among these are the Nürnberg Code (1947), the Helsinki Declaration (1964/1989) and the International Ethical Guidelines for Biomedical Research Involving Human Subjects, prepared by the Council for International Organizations of Medical Sciences (CIOMS), in cooperation with the World Health Organization (1982/1993). Three features in these documents are relevant to the questions you are raising. First of all, an important distinction is made between treatment and research, and some strong demands to be met are put forward concerning scientific experiments. Second, it is said that the benefit of the individual is

always to be given priority over that of research or society. Third, greater respect and harsher restrictions are expected the more defenceless and dependent each individual is in his or her environment.

These guidelines refer to the foetus and infant, not to fertilized eggs. Thus it cannot be deduced directly from these guidelines that fertilized eggs, which are the most dependent of all, deserve the most protection. Nevertheless, a long tradition challenges today's researchers with the following: if the principle of a specific obligation towards sick persons, children, the newly born, the unborn foetus is still considered valid, why is the scope of this principle limited so as not to include the most vulnerable of all — human life in its first weeks of life?

Ethical norms and values

You have also asked about the basis and standards which theology might contribute to your work in the form of relevant ethical norms.

We mentioned the most important element earlier, in our discussion of anthropology and its implications for actions vis-à-vis fertilized eggs. But we should now fill this out with reference to some central norms.

Your letter says that you and your colleagues regularly ask whether the work you carry out is of use to the group in question — in your case couples without children. You attach weight to the fact that the purpose shall be evident and significant. Apparently you reason that such a purpose gives ethical legitimation not only to research which does not destroy eggs but also to that which does.

This line of argumentation is familiar in the history of ethics as an ethics of usefulness or utilitarianism. In general, it maintains that an action is morally right if its consequences for humankind are better than those of other alternative actions. Such a consideration does satisfy important elements. Even theological ethics would evaluate positively a line of action that realizes values like health, welfare, freedom, justice.

A problem with utilitarian ethics is the weight given to one aspect while others are not taken into consideration. Therefore the so-called ethics of duty (also called deontological ethics) says that an action is right if attached to certain qualifications that meet certain given criteria. According to this kind of thinking, it is a duty to protect life, to tell the truth, not to steal and so forth. This way of thinking about norms is also supported by theological ethics (compare, for example, the ten commandments).

The research setting of which you are a part cannot be considered only from the perspective of usefulness. If all relevant norms are to be taken into account, we must also include elements of an ethics of duty. A key question is then the weight given to usefulness and duty respectively and how ethical norms from the two models can be balanced.

It is not surprising that the ethics of usefulness predominates in your work. In our opinion this reflects a cultural setting in which happiness and "the good life" form a central part both of the ideal of individuals and the goal for society. While this need not be wrong, it might lead us astray if it becomes the whole story. But what norms might be put forward as the foundation for a more complete and relevant consideration of dealing with fertilized eggs? Here we can only mention a few main elements.

Several values related to the ethics of consequence are relevant. Theological ethics will especially emphasize health, the evolving of life and community. These norms would have to be taken as valid when we consider the fertilized egg itself, both in the present and for the future, and the life-conditions of the parents. Viewed theologically, these norms are deeply rooted in the belief in God's good gifts of creation and the belief that human beings are created for community with fellow persons. While the understanding of health demands further explication (which we cannot go into here), it is necessary to nuance the definition of health as "complete physical, mental and social well-being" (World Health Organization). It is one thing to offer a utopian definition of health; it is quite another to idealize individual happiness and well-being in a way that does not give attention to the place of suffering in every human life. It would probably be reasonable to link the norm of "health" to the objective ability to function, but here we can do no more than suggest such a solution. "Evolving of life" expresses every human being's potential to realize the good and indwelling resources given in creation. The criterion of "community" points to the consideration that we are all part of large and small collectives and depend on each other in mutuality and joint responsibility.

A selection of norms of duty would also be of central value here. These are mainly to be understood as deduced from and rooted in the idea of human dignity. First and most important is the fifth commandment, which serves to protect biological existence itself. Luther and the Lutheran tradition have interpreted this commandment as a guard against all forms of violence and harm to the human body. Human dignity is concretized in the understanding of the equality of all, independent of gender, age, abilities or disabilities and the like. This norm offers an important corrective to any model of thought which ascribes weight to happiness and effectiveness. But we should mention further the duty to respect the personal integrity which is attributed to each human life. We believe this duty is significant as well for our attitude towards the unborn foetus and even fertilized eggs. As human life they have their "life space", with "borders" which should not be violated. Finally, theological ethics would put forward the imperative to care for the weak. According to the Bible, all human beings have a special responsibility to take care of the needy, poor and weak of different kinds through both a merciful attitude and actions of solidarity.

This range of norms offers a basis which might function constructively, given the main problems you raise in your letter. In concrete situations you might experience a conflict between what the norms of an ethics of consequence might support, and what the norms of an ethics of duty might demand. Ethical dilemmas like this cannot be solved in general; each must have an individual solution. Even so, it is important to know that some norms of an ethics of duty may count so heavily that no dispensation from them can be given in the name of advancing certain purposes or consequences. Thus, for instance, the right to life and integrity must be seen as protecting goods so fundamental to human beings that they cannot be violated even when the aim is to achieve a better evolving of life. Such norms mark the boundary for our choice of actions.

Some conclusions

Drawing on the premises we have just set forth, let us return briefly to some concrete problem areas within your field of work.

1. We both agree that research of a more clinical character on fertilized eggs which are to be brought back to the woman is

acceptable so long as the purpose is to give the egg increased possibilities to survive and develop into a living child. On an ethical basis, this purpose is satisfactory, and no fundamental norms of an ethics of duty are violated. However, this conclusion assumes that we accept IVF as ethically legitimate when certain conditions are met (which we cannot unfold here). We are aware that the method of IVF often implies that some fertilized eggs will have to be destroyed. It is important to find a method without "surplus eggs".

Our attitude is ambiguous towards the possibility of freezing and thawing fertilized eggs to try to make a childless woman pregnant. On the one hand, there are practical advantages in relation to the childless couple and the health of persons involved. On the other hand, complicating factors may include prolongation of storage time to make another pregnancy possible: this makes the question of society's use of resources with regard to reproductive technology of immediate interest. Even though a second child by IVF is much cheaper than the first, it could also lead to birth of two-egged twins born at different times. The main problem is that freezing and thawing fertilized eggs cannot be done today without destroying eggs by the mechanical damage by ice. From the perspective of an ethics of consequence, freezing must therefore be evaluated together with other forms of destroying eggs.

2. As to the different types of research in which eggs are destroyed, our conclusions diverge.

As mentioned, Anne-Marie believes that research on fertilized eggs should not be permitted, but accepts within a time limit of a fortnight exceptions under certain conditions. The time limit is motivated by the exceptional situation in which the just claims for the human value of the human fertilized egg must yield in a conflict between different evaluations. She suggests the following as an ethical norm: since fertilized human eggs are human personal life-in-becoming, with a rightful claim to human value, medical experimentation with them is not in general morally acceptable. Exceptions may be made within 14 days after fertilization (not counting any period during which they are frozen) only if all the following conditions are met: that such research aims at an improvement of the life process, that the insights gained are necessary and not otherwise available, that the donors of eggs and sperm have given their permission.

Lars maintains that all kinds of research in which eggs are destroyed are ethically impermissible. Such purposes and consequences as methodological improvements, increased embryological knowledge or pre-implantation diagnosis are not weighty enough to legitimate violation of certain fundamental norms of duty: the human being's right to life, respect of integrity and protection for the weak. Such actions are conclusively a violation of the dignity of human life in its earliest phase. Even useful consequences for parents, researchers or society cannot reduce a human life to an instrument for such purposes. Lars thus supports the idea that research which destroys fertilized eggs should be forbidden. This also includes an ethical critique of research aimed at developing a method for pre-implantation diagnosis.

All that remains is to say thank you for your interest in listening at some length to our thoughts. We eagerly await your reaction and comments. If it is possible for us to visit your institution, we might learn more about the questions you are faced with. Then together we could continue our dialogue

Regards,
Anne-Marie and Lars

6. *Euthanasia*

A Letter to a Nurse on Death and Dying

SVEND ANDERSEN and JAANA HALLAMAA

Dear Anne,

Thank you so much for your letter. It reminded me of the long and lively discussions we used to have while we were in nursing school about different problems, both theoretical and practical, that were brought up in our classes. Your letter made me realize how much I miss those talks. We did not count the hours or pay attention to the time of day (or night) when we plunged into the ethical dilemmas that we felt were raised so acutely by our future profession. I remember how we tried to consider the problems through our understanding of ourselves as Christians, called to serve God and our neighbour, and against the background of our own Lutheran tradition.

I was interested to learn from your letter that you have taken a new job in a nursing home. Working with elderly people who are in the last period of their lives is certainly quite different from your former work at the cancer unit or in the children's ward where you began right after our studies. As you say, you now face a new form of suffering, quite different from what you have been accustomed to in your former jobs, and a novel set of ethical dilemmas.

You mention the public debate about the end of life, the demand for a dignified death and the "right to die", and ask if I — after working with terminally ill patients for many years — have an opinion on these issues. You are correct in supposing that I often find my mind occupied with these problems. I am certainly willing to share some of my thoughts with you, and I hope we can then start a discussion in which we can help each other to discern better what is at stake here and what we as nurses and Christians should be thinking and doing.

The meaning of euthanasia

The demand for assistance to have one's life ended is frequently heard in the health care system, at least in the rich part of the world. In a way, this demand is an outcome of the culture and life-style of this part of the world where medical knowledge and improved means of treatment have made it possible to save many patients who in former times would have died. Improved life conditions mean that people live longer. The main causes of death are different from what they were some decades ago: fewer people die of infectious diseases and many more now die of cancer and cardiovascular diseases. This means that an increasing number of people have to go through extreme pain, deep fear and loss of mental abilities or consciousness before dying. Many people facing the prospect of unbearable pain or permanent unconsciousness wish that their doctor, instead of continuing a hopeless treatment, would bring their life to a painless end.

What these people are asking for is often called euthanasia. Literally, the word means "good death", though it is often associated with the practice in Nazi Germany of exterminating disabled people on the basis that their lives were "unworthy". In the current debate, however, euthanasia normally refers to a medical action performed by health care professionals with the purpose of ending a patient's life.

Some people distinguish "active" and "passive" euthanasia. The latter term is used for cases in which a patient's life is shortened by withdrawing or refraining from treatment that is very unlikely to bring any help to him or her. For example, in our nursing home we do not use intensive means to treat cases of pneumonia, because all our patients are terminally ill and such treatment would not improve their condition but would simply increase or prolong their sufferings. I would not call these cases euthanasia, even passive euthanasia, for the term seems to me to give the wrong impression that medicine could in these cases actually have control over the hour of death. What we really mean when we speak of passive euthanasia, then, is that we acknowledge the reality of death and give way to it without prolonging by medical means the process of the disease leading to death.

Euthanasia proper, or active euthanasia, is an intervention — such as a lethal injection — which directly causes a person's death. In some cases, however, this definition is problematic. If a patient is in severe pain and the alleviation of it requires a pain-killer so strong or a dose so large that death is hastened, is this euthanasia? In such cases, giving the medicine has a double effect — the relief of pain and the hastening of death — but only the first of these is intended. According to most moral theorists, a pre-known but unintended negative effect of an act is not morally incriminating (1) if the deed itself is morally good or at least morally neutral, (2) if it is done with good intention, and (3) if the other, intended effects of the deed are good.

There is another case that must be distinguished from euthanasia: a situation in which a patient wishes to kill herself or himself but is unable for one reason or another to do that and so asks a health care person to assist in suicide.

Traditionally, all penal codes have classified both active euthanasia and assisting in suicide as crimes, either murder or manslaughter. But many people today do not consider euthanasia or assistance in suicide as crimes. They believe this is something that should be legally available to people who wish to die. In the Netherlands euthanasia and assisted suicide are no longer regarded as acts of homicide. The Dutch parliament has decided that a doctor who declares that the death of a patient was caused by euthanasia or assisted suicide will not be prosecuted if the following conditions are fulfilled:

— the patient had repeatedly requested euthanasia;
— before death, the patient was in a medically hopeless situation without any prospects of recovery;
— the doctor had consulted with a colleague about the diagnosis and the prognosis;
— the doctor is in a position to produce a report on all relevant medical facts about the disease of which the patient was dying.

Towards a Christian approach

Many people regard the Dutch solution, although regulated by law, as problematic. They see it as preparing the way for disrespect towards "hopeless" cases and as a sign of fear in the face of suffering. But what should we as Christians think about euthanasia?

We miss the point if we think the ethical question concerning euthanasia is simply: "Is it permissible to kill another human being?" There are at least two questions involved: "Can it be legitimate for a human being to prefer death to life?" and "Is it permissible to end another person's life if she or he wishes to die?" Furthermore, there are also two distinct perspectives from which we have to consider the issue — as individual Christians and as members of a social community and society.

All of us must face death as individual human persons. From this point of view, death is not just an ethical issue. On the contrary, traditional Lutheran vocabulary calls death a spiritual matter: it is something in which our relationship to God is at stake. So the most important question is whether our faith survives the prospect of death. Agony in the face of death is not a sign of a fight for survival but of a fight against despair that threatens to destroy the trusting faith.

If we consider death from the spiritual point of view, is it not obvious that the wish to be relieved from pain must simply be condemned? Is it not a manifestation of self-assertion, of claiming a right against God? Many Christians ask questions like these in connection with euthanasia. But we should see that there are other equally important questions, such as: If the wish to die springs from the experience that life has come to an end, is it not incessant treatment rather than the wish to die that manifests human self-assertion and reluctance to accept the finitude of life?

We cannot hope to dispose of these questions by somehow finding a clear and certain answer to them from a detached theoretical position. These are questions which are deeply human in the sense that they concern every one of us and in the sense that we cannot come to a definite and final conclusion about them. No, death and dying — and thus euthanasia — will continue to perplex us as long as we live. Psychologically, it would be easier to fix a definite answer for all times and places, and understandably there are many people who wish to do that. I do not think that this accords with a Lutheran understanding of the moral responsibility of the human person. We must always remain ethically alert, not pretending to have found a final answer to our questions and not condemning people who have arrived at a moral conclusion we ourselves do not accept.

If we see the question of death in the broad perspective of the Christian faith, the wish to die can be wholly legitimate. This does not solve the problem of euthanasia, but we can still ask whether all cases of euthanasia are violations of the fifth commandment. The prohibition of killing has never been obeyed without exceptions. Christians have accepted capital punishment; they have killed in wars and in self-defence. Moreover, the ten commandments on the Lutheran understanding are not absolute moral norms as such but absolute only as a manifestation of the double commandment to love God more than anything and our neighbours as ourselves (Matthew 22:37-40). The question is then whether it is possible that love sometimes requires actively assisting someone to die. This is a difficult question, and I do not think that we can give a definite answer to it, covering all times and places, every situation and circumstance. Even if we concluded that there is no absolute and general No to euthanasia on the basis of the Christian faith, this conclusion cannot be extended to the societal sphere, for to do so would mean that health care professionals, like you and me, would be entitled and even obliged to perform euthanasia and assist in suicide in an authorized way. Such legitimation cannot be based on Christian ethics as we understand it.

When we consider euthanasia in the social sphere, we are no longer talking about the individual acts of private persons in unique situations. Rather, we are considering the arrangement of institutions — in our case the health care system — and the routine acts performed by professionals within these institutions. In traditional Lutheran language, we are talking about "worldly orders" and corresponding callings.

The institution of health care systems takes shape according to the ethical thinking which influences their organization. All social institutions, health care included, should be based on the ethics of the Golden Rule as the secular rational counterpart of Christian neighbourly love. This means that a health care system should fulfil the requirements of beneficence — by securing treatment of diseases and illness — and distributive justice — by ensuring equal access for all citizens to proper medical treatment.

But these general considerations do not answer the question whether active euthanasia should be legally introduced into the health care system. As some people see it, the demand of beneficence gives a patient the right to have his or her life ended at will by health care professionals, and euthanasia should thus be legalized as a part of the health care system. But would such legislation accord with the ethical principles on which the health care system is founded? The specific kind of beneficence health care professionals traditionally show — helping people to survive, curing them, caring for them — is fundamentally life-furthering. How can one reconcile this traditional interpretation of beneficence with an understanding which would involve actively ending a patient's life? Accordingly, we as Christians cannot favour legislation which explicitly gives health care professionals permission to kill their patients or even obliges them to do so. No law can legitimately make it a part of one's professional task to use killing as a means to fight human suffering. Thus the practice of euthanasia cannot be accepted as a part of the legitimate "worldly order".

Working with suffering patients

As nurses we face the problem of euthanasia from two different perspectives, and this sometimes makes the question even more difficult than it would otherwise be. We are human persons who think and feel, who suffer when we have to see other people suffer. But we are also professionals who have a regulated function to fulfil within an institution. What can we then do?

Let me tell you something about my own experience. Only after having worked for several years with terminally ill patients did I realize that a great deal of the anguish I had felt for my patients — having to see their suffering — was caused by my own fear of pain and death and by my feeling of powerlessness. I was constantly trying to find technical and medical means to make my patients feel better rather than simply being present as a fellow human person with them in their suffering. It took me a long time to recognize my own fear and my feelings of inadequacy and powerlessness. I came to realize that the image I had fostered of myself as a nurse bore features of omnipotence — the idea that I as a nurse should be in control of everything that my patients have to go through. It was difficult to give up this idea of omnipotence, but it was also a great relief.

I still find it hard to see other people suffer. I still find it hard to accept that we medical professionals cannot control life and death. But

I also think that I have found some positive ways, both professional and private, to cope with my anguish. I now work in a society whose purpose is to further palliative care. I have become acquainted with the ideas of hospices, special homes for dying patients. I hope in this way to develop myself as a nurse for the benefit of my patients. There are, naturally, other ways of achieving the same end.

My private means of enduring the pressure of my work involve leading an ordinary life as a Christian in a Christian community. There I have come to realize that I do not have to solve the problem of suffering; I cannot do that. I do not even have to try to show people that there is a meaning behind their suffering, because I cannot do that either. As a Christian I am in the hospital to fulfil my calling as a nurse by doing my work as well as possible and living under the mercy of God in the service of other people. It is in this way, I am certain, that God works in our world.

I look forward to hearing from you soon.

Sincerely yours,
Jane

7. *Justice, Dignity, Autonomy*

A Letter to an Old Friend on the Quality of Life

JUKKA-MIKKO KARJALAINEN

Dear Robert,

Since we met some time ago, I have been thinking about our conversation. When you told me how old you are I could hardly believe it — and you said yourself that you are feeling quite young. But many of your friends have already died and many of the others are beginning to be ill much more often than before. So, you said, you have begun to think about the moral problems in health care which you and perhaps your relatives might confront sooner or later.

Let me tell you about an interesting meeting to which I was invited recently as a representative of the Lutheran church. The board of directors of a large community hospital was talking over the priority guidelines for patient selection in internal medicine and surgery. They also had a secondary task: to discuss the principles according to which patients should be cared for and treated in situations at the end of life.

To be more practical, they had chosen an enlightening case study for discussion. The case was as follows. There are two patients on an internal medicine ward waiting for a new liver. One is a woman teacher, a 72-year-old widow who has been in good health except for a quite recently discovered severe liver dysfunction. Until now she has been very active socially. She has four children and twelve grandchildren, three of whom have enjoyed her "day-care" because of the shortage of facilities in the community.

The other patient is a 23-year-old man who has been studying philosophy and linguistics at the university for three years. His wife is pregnant. His life was good before he was taken to hospital, and his health problem is the same as the teacher's. Both have a reasonable prognosis if a proper liver can be supplied. Their blood types and other medical qualifications are unfortunately alike. Consequently, the caring team is asked to give reasons for choosing one or the other of the two persons for the remedy if only one liver is available for transplant.

As you can imagine, the board's discussion of this was intensive. The board members' main concerns were the proportionately diminishing capacity of the health-care system to meet the needs of the ageing population and the allocation of medical resources. A secondary concern was the right to self-determination and to human dignity at the end of life. Some answers were found, but many of the issues remained unresolved. It would be interesting to hear your reaction to some of the points that emerged in the discussion.

The meaning of old age

One of the most difficult problems discussed was whether the age of the patient has any bearing on ethical reasoning and judgments — and if so, why? It was apparent that it is not easy to talk about this. Age is a relative and sometimes quite sensitive matter. In many cultures it is considered impolite to ask the age of an adult, because age as such is somehow something a person may be ashamed of. Furthermore, in the same community old people may in one respect be highly esteemed because of their life experience and in another respect considered at the same time to be an economic burden. Most old people do not have paid employment, so they may become a burden to those who work. But if they were to continue working, it would mean that a number of younger citizens would be unemployed. Because of the sensitive nature of these ideas, they are often avoided or concealed in everyday talk and action.

Perhaps the basic problem in discussing age is the matter of point of view. Most of us know our own age exactly (though some people do not), but it is a commonplace to say that a person is "only as old as he or she feels". Simultaneously feeling young and being old seems not to be contradictory. Besides calendar years, age is thus also a matter of a person's own experience and sentiments. This experience is made up of many psychological, social, cultural and other environmental factors. The woman referred to earlier, for example, has had an opportunity to take care of her grandchildren, which has perhaps been one of her motivations for living and thus for taking care of herself.

Old age can be analyzed by different branches of science, yet what it really means to be old is very hard to define without making a normative judgment. So when does a person become old? If it were only a question of time and chronology, as the word "when" seems to indicate, people would become old when they reached a certain number of years of life. Even so, the question would arise of what number that is. For all practical purposes, the maximum life span of a human person is about 100 years, but relatively few people in fact attain that age. Should old age then depend, for example, on the average life-span in a given community? The man of 23 thinks the woman of 72 is old, but someone at 95 would say she is young.

Others might suggest that old age depends on certain changes in one's appearance and physical and mental capabilities which we can discern as time goes by. But such changes are not necessarily bound to a person's years of life. Diminishing physical strength, grey hair, baldness and wrinkles are not necessarily signs of ageing. Nor can old age be defined by assessing psychological matters like one's attitude to life. Young people can often be more conservative or pessimistic than their grandparents. Still, it is true that in most cases others assess a person's age only by looking at the external signs of ageing, as above, which may in some cases be totally misleading.

If the number of years of life as such is hard to take as the decisive factor in allocating medical resources, the answer must depend on the changes which take place in the ageing persons and, accordingly, the differences between older and younger persons and the characteristics of persons or groups of persons at different ages.

By what can old people then be clearly distinguished as a group from the middle-aged and even younger? Several common images can of course be cited: old people are socially isolated or neglected by their families, most old people have poor health, old people are not interested in sex, old people are unable to learn new things and intelligence decreases as one becomes older, they do not have strength enough to work, they have no political power or influence.

Behind all the stereotypes lies the assumption that all old people are alike. In fact the opposite is true: individual differences among people increase with age. So these common beliefs are misconceptions. The social isolation of old people is not a fact. Most old people do not live alone, nor do they feel lonely. Some of them voluntarily choose to live alone. Of course, it is a fact that the older a person becomes the fewer of his or her relatives, friends and acquaintances are alive. It is also a fact that there is a growing disproportion between men and women among the older age groups. Because women live longer than men, the ratio of women to men is higher among older people. But old age, possible social isolation and disproportionality between sexes are not medical problems. Why then should these factors have something to do with the fair distribution of medical resources?

Although morbidity increases as people become older, not all of the elderly are in poor health. Old people can enjoy sex, too, while at the same time some experience their lives as being easier without sex. Old people are not unable to learn, nor does their intelligence decrease. Old people are not politically powerless; indeed, their increasing numbers may give them more political influence.

However, all these false claims and stereotypes can find their way into moral reasoning, though this may be concealed behind the attitudes of the decision-makers. And the upshot of all these misconceptions may be conclusions like the following: life is without purpose and meaningless when you become old; you need not live if you are old; your interests need not be taken into account in ethical reasoning.

A great number of things thus speak against the idea that the age of a person is an ethically relevant factor or should be decisive. Age is a relative matter, and decisions should be based on norms which are in fact only statistical averages. From the individual point of view these statistics may lead to dangerous fallacies. Old people are no more alike than young people. Thus, the principle that scarce medical resources should be allocated only according to the expected life-span of the patient must be rejected.

Principles of justice

But do we not have enough information about the persons in the case above? We know them; they are not statistics. The old teacher and the young student are not alike in every respect. Why would we not use some well-known, common and general principles of justice? For example:

1. To each according to his or her needs. The principle of need is very important in the allocation of medical resources; the basic task of health care is to meet the manifold needs of the sick and suffering. This principle guides us to direct remedies primarily to those who suffer from the most serious injuries or who are in the greatest distress. Usually, if health needs are not met, the result will be some permanent deficiency or failure of bodily or other functions. Accordingly, needs must be distinguished from interests and desires or wishes. Still, in many cases the needs too are various. In the case we are looking at, the needs are clear: both patients will die before long if their need for a new liver is not met. So the problem with using the principle of need in this case is that the persons have similar needs. The principle of need is quite useless if the needs of both parties are similar and equally strong. But are they in fact equally strong? Could the need for a new liver be transformed into the need to get more years to live? If so, could it be argued that the need of a 72-year-old teacher is less than that of a 23-year-old student, because the former is expected to have less time left to live than the latter, all other things being equal? But the argument that the young man's need for more years of life is stronger seems absurd. So we have to try to apply some other principles.

2. To each according to his or her merits. According to this principle, social and other services should be distributed primarily to those who have done something praiseworthy or favourable. This norm, which can be called the principle of merit, links access to health care services to an individual's actions and life-style. The old woman no doubt has a good deal of merit which one can identify. She has probably paid a great sum in taxes over her life, for example; and a liver transplant is quite a costly operation. Why should she not be granted a service for which she has in a sense paid in advance? She has reared and helped to rear a number of good citizens; and her service as a teacher must surely be appreciated as a service to society. Should not the community repay its "spiritual" and social debt to her? She may also have had a healthy way of life; she has been a non-smoker and non-drinker and has never taken unnecessary health risks. Her troublesome fate is in no sense self-inflicted. Assuming these circumstances and merits, why should she — or anyone else in a similar position — not merit compensation in the form of a new liver?

While it may seem to us that all these "good deeds" deserve recompense, and that individuals derive certain rights from certain praiseworthy performances, from the ethical point of view we must take the entire situation into account. And this woman is not alone in her distress. The student is her fellow-sufferer. We have already seen that the needs of both persons are alike. But are their merits? It surely seems possible on the face of it to compare their lives in this respect. Perhaps we will discover that the student has also lived a respectable and healthy life, which could be considered meritorious. Yet it will be difficult to prove that he deserves anything on the basis of his career — because he has not yet had one. In the area of work, he is less meritorious than the teacher. But would it really be fair to give priority to the teacher given that the young student at 23 has not had the chance to earn any merit through his work? Perhaps we should thus try to calculate their "merit" in proportion to the opportunities they have had due to their age.

It is evident that the problems of trying to make such calculations in order to apply the principle of merit to health care are insuperable. First of all, we should have to agree on what kinds of merit are relevant to the distribution of health care-services. No such consensus exists. Should we take into account only the so-called health-related factors, such as life-styles? How do we distinguish contingencies from things which have happened inevitably?

As this case study shows, it is troublesome and even painful to compare the merits of two persons or groups of persons just because of their difference in age. Too much is left to the imagination, and thus is prone to error. There are too many unknown factors. If we could reliably find out the merits of each individual, we could confront the problem of measuring them. The vocation of physicians and nurses is to cure and care. Whose task should it be to weigh and measure merits?

The distribution of scarce medical resources cannot be based only on merits any more than on needs. The principle of merit is not in itself dangerous. The danger lies in one of the characteristics of human nature: the inclination to reward, to avenge and to punish. This tendency is especially prominent in critical social situations and times of transition. If this is forgotten, the distribution of the rewards and punishments will no longer be based on clear facts and principles.

The principle of merit is closely linked to the idea that individuals must in the end cope with the tragedies of their lives by themselves. This pattern of thought is contrary to the Christian belief in mercy, forgiveness and love for one's neighbour. Forgiveness and mercy need no reasons or explanations. They are gifts.

3. To each according to his or her contribution to society. According to this principle some people are entitled to something because they are contributing or will contribute more to society than some others. Their contribution may be of a variety of types. Yet what is to be assessed are the presumed good or bad consequences of the choice. Of course, nearly any moral reflection resulting in a moral judgment will take into account the good and the evil produced. But what is to be considered good or evil for society in each case — and specifically in the case I have been discussing? Should the liver be given to the person who is likely to become the more economically productive member of the society? For example, would a healthy taxpayer be considered a good investment and a pensioner who, though healthy, is using up resources from the social welfare budget, a bad one? Since the life-expectancy of the young man is most likely longer than that of the old teacher, the cost-benefit calculus with respect to society as a whole would speak in favour of giving the liver to him.

But just as the principle of merit runs up against difficulties of determining the real merits of each person, so the principle of contribution to society proves doubtful because of the difficulties in predicting the social consequences of the choices made. The young man might rear a new family, work hard and make his wife and children happy. But what if he suddenly decides to lead a life of comfort or even indulgence at the expense of his wife, relatives or society? Or what if he remains unemployed? The old teacher has been an exemplary person; she may still continue to take care of her grandchildren and provide an ideal model of loving humaneness to the younger generation — and so even help to break down the stereotypes about old people prevailing in her immediate context.

What would then be the cost of choosing one or the other? Life for one, sorrow and grief for the other. No matter which choice we made, it would also have negative consequences. If the aggregate of the good consequences of either choice is equal to the other, what should be done? Should a decision be made by lottery? If so, how should the "loser" be treated? Does society owe him or her something? Would it be right also to impose some obligations on the winner?

The foregoing reasoning may sound cruel, at least in its application. It means that both persons were being used as means to achieve a social end. The one who did not get the liver would be used *only* as a means. The other would also be used as a means, but as the recipient of the life-saving liver would probably feel as though he or she were being treated as an end. So would it be wrong to base the choice on the impression (it cannot be based on pure facts) of the contribution of the person to society? Surely their human dignity is at stake and must be respected, though it is very difficult to tell how human dignity obligates us. However, its practical meaning can be seen, for example, when the person's will is respected and when the person's existence is valued above economic interests.

4. To each according to the principles of the free market. Although the health-care systems in most Western European countries, for example, are primarily funded by governmental budgets, there are still some services that are supplied more or less according to the principles of the free market. Obviously it would be possible to establish a system distributing health care chiefly according to this principle, but would it be just and fair? Such a health-care system would operate primarily according to the law of supply and demand. Since people will certainly always have health needs, the demand will always exist. The problem is of course that those in need are not necessarily those who have enough money to buy the available services. Consequently, the health-care system would concentrate on patients who can afford to "buy health". This would lead to serious problems of inequality in other respects. Morbidity is bound to social factors; it is more common in the lower social and economic strata than in the higher. It is also statistically bound to age. Young people tend to be healthier than old people, and although older people are statistically wealthier than the younger, the individual differences are great. Imagine that the final choice in our case were made on grounds of the wealth of one or the other of the two persons. Given that the wealth of persons may depend entirely on accidental factors (fortunate investments, inheritance, lottery prizes), it is clear that allocating treatment according to the principles of the free market cannot be fair, nor indeed is it the way most of us would expect.

5. To each according to the established expectations of his or her society. While this principle is on the face of it obvious, the question of what are the established expectations, for example, towards the welfare services is a sociological one. They could possibly be studied. After all, the moral question would remain: are the attitudes and values morally defensible and fair? They would probably consist of a set of principles such as we are discussing here. What is the right weight to be given to each norm, principle or value? This weighting should be an ongoing process, because the circumstances will vary from time to time. Thus, the weighting will be more difficult in times of great social change, such as the rapid growth in the proportion of old people in the population of Western countries. Moreover, it would probably be easier for citizens to accept the distribution of treatment according to a certain set of material principles of justice if they were more aware of the principles themselves and better informed about the problems in health care and how health-care systems work. The problem of justice in health care can be seen as partly educational in nature, and not just as a dispute concerning the claims or rights of, for example, the younger and older generations.

The problem of distributive justice is also a methodological one: how do we agree on the principles we are willing to follow? Could there be a new "social contract", according to which the scarce resources would be allocated? While this question is of great theoretical interest, in practice we will have to be content for the present with the prevailing democratic and legislative systems. And although the real choices have to be made within legal premises, the problem of fair allocation is impossible to solve by purely legislative means.

But it would seem that our case is not only a matter of justice. The principle of beneficence and the right of self-determination could also be applied to it. The teacher might have an altruistic attitude towards the young student. How should we react if she voluntarily wanted to give up the possibility of receiving the liver transplant, to which she might be entitled? Does she have the right to do as she likes with her own life? Would such an act manifest the deepest possible respect and love for another person's life and dignity? Or, if her motive was the egoistical one of avoiding her own future pain, would she in that way be showing disrespect towards her own gift of life and her own dignity as a person?

The meanings of dignity

The concept of dignity itself is of great importance. It has several aspects, and an entire ethical system can be based on the concept of human dignity.

The most important implication of the notion of human dignity is the equality of human persons. It would be unjust and a violation of human dignity if persons needing similar care were treated differently without proper reasons. All people are equal because of their equal dignity. The dignity of human beings is based on their creation in God's image and on the love of Christ, which belong to everyone. Therefore, human dignity does not depend on a person's characteristics — age, contribution to society, health, abilities or disabilities, virtue or vice. And because dignity belongs to the human being by creation, it can never be lost.

However, human dignity is not without ambiguity. For example, it can be seen as a justification for not interfering with a person's freedom as well as a justification for helping the needy even without their consent. The apparent contradiction here can be explained as follows: on the one hand, human dignity implies the integrity of the person; on the other, it implies his or her physical well-being, based on the values of life and health. As created by God, the human person is an individual, and this individuality is dignified by protecting his or her personal freedom. But there are also other values, like life and health, which can or must be protected. Protecting these values may sometimes require certain constraints on individual freedom. But the ultimate ground for the protection of these values is the person's human dignity; his or her dignity as a human being is protected by restricting his or her possibilities to act or to do something to himself or herself. Thus the basic norm of human dignity can be used as a justification for different kinds of activities.

The dignity of a person can be distinguished from his or her human dignity. It is possible to violate and even lose one's dignity as a person by acting against one's conscience or against principles one knows are right, or by continuously destroying one's life, or by building one's affairs on lies; even so, one does not thereby lose one's human dignity.

Applying this to our case, imagine that one or another of the patients — say, the teacher — would refuse the treatment. We might then ask whether the old woman would lose her dignity as a person if she voluntarily gave up her chance of getting the liver? To answer yes would be the same as to say that she did wrong — in other words, we would be admitting that it is wrong to sacrifice one's life for another person. Would her human dignity and right of self-determination be violated if she were *not* allowed to give up her chance of getting the liver? Would it be wrong not to permit the old woman to benefit the young student? Perhaps she could be acting on purely altruistic grounds. She might have her reason to live, but would like in this desperate situation to give the chance to the young man. This would not mean an immediate end to her own life. She could be treated and cared for well, although not cured. Her own will would be taken into account. She would not need to suffer from a violation or loss of human dignity. The medical and nursing staff would avoid having to make a painful decision.

Does my life belong to me?

It may happen — as the old teacher perhaps fears — that life itself becomes unbearable. In such a situation one might ask, "Does my life not belong to me? Do I not have a right to give up my life? To whom does my life in principle belong?"

The expression "my life" seems to be quite clear: if I am a living person, the life I am living is possessed by myself. However, if we believe that we are created by God, we consider that our lives are a gift from God. Several questions then arise. Does the gift of life become the property of the recipient? Is not everything that is given or made by God somehow sacred? Does the sacredness of human life mean that it must be left untouched? Does this mean that only God is justified in "making decisions" on human life?

But even if life is a gift from God, it is clear that dying and death are necessary parts of that gift. If we have a right to the life which has been given, does that right imply a right to die? Or if everyone must of necessity die, is it somehow absurd to speak of a "right to die"? It should be remembered that although we can to some degree choose our life-styles, only a minority of people really have the opportunity to choose their way of dying. At the same time, if we have the right to a good or decent life, why should we not have the right to a good or easy death? But what kind of death is a *good* death? Since death and dying are parts of one's life, the answer to this question depends mostly on one's idea of what a good life is, as well as the situation at a particular time.

In what kinds of situations is it sensible to ask questions like these? In other words, why do we talk about *easy* ways of dying? The word "easy" in this context clearly seems to carry a negative connotation. But our notion of what is easy obviously depends on our conception of what is difficult. What would be the "difficult" way out? Could we imagine a harder way to die than one that is long, seemingly endless, full of pain and suffering and which we have to walk alone? Do we have a right to restrain a person from departing life with dignity and as restfully as possible?

The purpose of human life cannot be suffering, not even at its end. No one should be prohibited if for some reason he or she wants to suffer. Nevertheless, it would be very peculiar to prevent someone from making his or her life as pleasant and comfortable as possible, so long as this does not harm others. That is to say, life is also a matter of *quality*. But what then are the basic components of a good life? Of what sorts of things is human well-being constituted?

The value of autonomy and the quality of life

Perhaps you have thought often about what kind of life is good or what things and circumstances would make you happy. The first among the general factors one could mention as conditions for human life to be of good quality is the fulfilment of the basic needs; indeed life cannot exist at all where basic human needs are not met. Closely related is a second condition, health; while it is not easy to define, it is clearly more than just the absence of certain handicaps or symptoms of disease like pain and suffering. Third, one ought to have a sphere of personal freedom. A person who has at least some basic choices can make his or her life meaningful. A fourth element of the quality of life could be a person's social relations — that he or she can love and be loved. Fifth, it is said that a person ought to have some purpose, some reason to feel that his or her life is meaningful. Life without any goals to aim at feels empty. The purpose of life consists of the set of one's own values, norms, principles and appreciations. These are on the one hand a part of morality and on the other hand a framework for assessing the quality of life.

It is not easy in individual cases to assess what kind of life is of good quality. The conditions listed above may have varying importance to different persons at different ages, but should they be given an overall order of priority?

The place of personal freedom is one of the trickiest questions in ranking the conditions for a human life of good quality. Should we prefer freedom to health, for example? To give a definite answer is difficult not only because of the vagueness of what is meant by the value of freedom but also because of factual and empirical issues that bear on human freedom. On the whole, we should be able to agree on the constitutive elements of freedom. Roughly speaking, it can be said that to be autonomous or free means that one can do, act or omit. To say that a person *can* do or not do something is equivalent to saying that he or she has ability and opportunity. Ability refers to the internal preconditions of an act and opportunity to its external preconditions.

To come back to our case study, do these two persons have the mental capacities to make a clear and unambiguous decision? Do they have sufficient external possibilities to follow through the consequences of their own choices? If the answer is yes, it will be difficult to find arguments against their own decisions. Yet it must be remembered also that freedom is relative in the sense that a person may be able to make choices in some respects and unable in other respects. The old teacher and the young student are in a very critical situation regarding their freedom and well-being. Surely, if possible, their well-being should be ensured so that they could make a free choice.

Why then should individual freedom be so highly respected a value? The answer is based on the meanings of freedom to human beings. The first meaning perhaps lies in the fact that freedom gives a person the possibilities to live as he or she likes, to carry out his or her interests, to make dreams come true. Freedom gives power and joy in life. It is one of the preconditions of happiness and thus one of the factors contributing to the quality of life. On this understanding the notion of freedom may seem quite idealistic and sometimes unreal. Illness can surprise and ideals be wrecked. Nevertheless, in the midst of everything, ideals are the source of life and hope. Second, autonomy also has clearly ethical implications. Human freedom is a presupposition for a person's being responsible. Only a free person can have duties. Yet the primary value of autonomy for human beings seems to rest upon the first of its meanings.

But answering the question of the value of autonomy gives rise to further questions. Does the value of life depend on the value and the quantity of autonomy? Is the quality of life more important than the quantity? Do old people prefer safety and well-being to freedom? What should they prefer? What are the consequences of a person's experience of his or her own health for his or her preferences? Although old age may diminish physical strength and bring about a variety of complaints, an older person may at the same time get new dimensions and different opportunities from what he or she formerly had. These depend of course on the person's internal as well as external conditions, such as health, social relations and economic standing.

Living wills and the willingness to live

It may happen that patients are temporarily unable to express their own wishes or that they sink into a deep and irreversible coma. This is why many people think of preparing a "living will", expressing the person's own request not to be kept alive in a situation where there is no reasonable hope of recovery from a physical or mental disability. Normally it is a written document stating the person's own wishes and signed by the person and a couple of witnesses.

The main aims of a living will are to enhance individual self-determination, to avoid unnecessary suffering and to facilitate decision-making at the end of life. Yet a living will can also be signed from a purely altruistic point of view. Although it would be a useful practice, we do not have a duty to announce in advance our will concerning the last days of our lives.

Living wills are not without problems, of which at least three should be mentioned. Their legal status in some countries is unclear. Since a living will can be prepared at any time after a person has reached majority, its reliability may become questionable, particularly if there is a long lapse of time between the signing and the onset of the person's terminal condition. Living wills may also be vague in the sense that it is impossible to anticipate and describe in advance all kinds of situations that may arise.

The fact is that life itself cannot be described in advance, not even for the immediate future. Life cannot be predicted. Life is a gift and a riddle, which we may try to solve, but with no guarantee that we can. Its length is not wholly in our hands. Ageing is inevitable, but it must not be seen only in terms of problems. It is also full of possibilities. Not all problems can be resolved by developing new medicines and new therapeutic measures: and if such remedies could be invented, they would hardly be accessible to all. Life has its limits.

Life, ageing and old age cannot be resolved even by setting principles, values or norms, whether moral or legal. Principles alone are not enough; they must also be followed. Unfortunately, that is not always so easy. Cases and situations may prove troublesome and people may be selfish or nonchalant. If possible, the minimum we ought to do is to try to live in real time and to be informed about facts and principles. Whether young or old, the maximum we can do is to grasp life — if possible now!

Regards,
Your friend, Paul

8. *Legislation on Human and Animal Research*

A Letter to a Parliamentarian

GERT NILSSON and HANS-OLOF KVIST

Dear Member of Parliament,

Thank you for your recent letter, in which you ask how we as members of your congregation regard some of the current issues related to genetic research, biotechnology and medical technology about which the legislature may soon have to make some decisions. We believe that it is part of the task of the church to bring to the fore values which we may not violate because of human dignity and the integrity of creation and to clarify conflicts of values in terms of current realities.

First of all, we want to emphasize that the church does not have a negative attitude towards new techniques as such. Quite the contrary. In our opinion, it is one of the vocations of the human being to manage and to develop nature in such a way that it can serve and give pleasure to human beings and other forms of life. We consider it unfortunate that some Christians regard biotechnology as interference with creation that should generally be forbidden. Christian tradition considers that one of the mandates given to human beings is to create culture and to search for the truth. Humankind uses the resources of creation to survive, and human history can help it to try to see the connections and plan the future.

This is not to say that nature derives its value from culture. On the contrary, nature has its own intrinsic value, which exists independently of its utility to human beings and must not be violated by human beings. It is not culture that provides nature with its value;

rather, nature is the condition for culture. The search for truth is connected to both nature and culture. In human beings there is a struggle and a longing to see and discover the physical connection as well as the metaphysical or religious connection.

This emphasis implies a great respect towards science and technical development, but as means for and not goals of the human being's way of life.

Having said this, we also want to emphasize that there are some limits to culture and to the search for truth. These limits are not primarily constituted by theological doctrines or political ideologies, but by life itself and by a respect for everything that is alive. We are well aware that the church has in the past sometimes wanted to control science and culture, just as political ideologies in the East and West have tried to do in more recent times. We want to distance ourselves from any such ideas which, we believe, violate the human being as a person. When we claim that research and culture are limited, we are referring to something else, namely, human dignity and the integrity of the whole creation. The dignity of the human being is more important than the freedom of research; respect for the integrity of the human being is more important than the development of technology. The sense of moral responsibility which is unique to humanity will help us to avoid certain ways and to discover others.

People sometimes defend the violation of the value of a few individuals in order to achieve the goal of improving the life of a large number of human beings. The premise of this argument is that the good has primacy over the right. We would like to emphasize the reverse principle, that the right stands before the good or, even better, that the right and the good walk hand in hand. To be able to do the right you must have a certain conception about the good, and to do the good you have to be guided by what is the right. Thus the principle that "the end justifies the means" can never be morally acceptable as an ethical principle.

As a guiding principle for biotechnology and medical technology we would insist that the dignity of the human being and its integrity constitute a limit in front of which science and technology must stop. But there is also another limit: the integrity of creation. The creation has an intrinsic value, not just an instrumental one. Human beings are allowed to use the creation for their survival and for their culture, but they are not permitted to destroy nature.

The development of knowledge and technology have reached the point where the genetic code can be manipulated by human beings. It is necessary to pause and ask what right we have as human beings to do such manipulations? Do we have the right to manipulate genes in order to breed extremely thin pigs for the convenience of human diets low in fat? Or cows who produce so much milk that their udders trail painfully along the ground? Do we have the right to produce synthetic cocoa biotechnologically and thereafter consider the cacao plant useless and let it disappear from the earth's flora?

Some would of course argue that there is a distinction between research and the development of technology, and that human beings should be free in their research work but regulated in the development of technology. One important argument for this position is that a society cannot force people not to think. Others would contend that society must have an ethic to guide researchers and politicians. Biotechnological research, after all, is not just done by abstract reasoning; it also depends on experiments carried out on human beings, animals and the creation.

Moreover, research and the development of technology go hand-in-hand, not least in the area of medical technology. By the time research in a given area has shown certain results, an application in which these results are used has already been established. Foetal diagnostics, artificial insemination and *in vitro* fertilization exemplify this. Heart transplants are another example. We can imagine a futuristic scenario in which it will be possible, by manipulating sex cells, to eliminate schizophrenia or to create élite sportsmen and sportswomen. In the discussions about anabolic steroids it has already been mentioned that performance-enhancing drugs will be superfluous in the future, when it will be possible to achieve the same effect permanently by gene manipulation. In our opinion, however, manipulating of sex cells is not possible.

In fact, biomedical research, experiments on human beings or fertilized eggs and development of new technology cannot be separated from each other; and it is of course impossible to create new medicines or methods of treatment without experiments. For this reason, we believe we must respect the limit set by the integrity, dignity and value of the human being. At the same time, one may ask what is best for human integrity — to let people live with incurable diseases or to experiment with therapies that give unreliable results in an indefinite time? The ethical debate has to take issues like this seriously.

A common argument in favour of free research and biotechnological development is that there are needs that have to be satisfied. But needs are very uncertain criteria for right and wrong, because needs can be created and they can arise because there are no alternatives.

According to the Christian view of the human being, the human person has a responsibility for himself or herself, for his or her fellow-beings and for the whole surrounding creation. A person has this responsibility towards the Creator. In a way it is this responsibility that marks out the specifically human, that differentiates human beings from animals. Responsibility has many nuances. Part of human responsibility is responsibility for what is done in the world and with the world, including one's fellow-beings; part of it is responsibility for using one's personal resources in a constructive way.

To want to go beyond the limits set by nature is a normal feature of human beings. Moral responsibility seeks to regulate this exceeding of the limits in order to safeguard the integrity of human beings, and not to violate the integrity of creation apart from clearly justifiable and exceptional cases.

With these few remarks on issues of principle, we now turn to some concrete problems.

Collection and keeping of human genetic information. The collection and storage of genetic information is primarily of interest for medical research, diagnostics and therapy. At the same time, there may be a demand for such data from insurance companies and employers. To prevent abuse of sensitive information, the handling of these data must be regulated by law. An indispensable condition is that the persons concerned must always give their permission if genetic information about them is to be kept. Information collected for a specific purpose may not be kept longer than necessary; when the aim is reached, the information should be destroyed.

Even so an abuse can strike the individual. For example, an insurance company may ask for genetic information about an individual, claiming that any client is entitled to decline to give it. Thus authorizing the information seems voluntary and sounds safe. In practice, however, refusing to give information can be interpreted as showing that the person has something to hide, and the consequence of such a refusal might be more unfavourable terms of coverage and higher premiums than if the information were provided.

Legislation should be worked out in such a way that genetic information cannot be used outside the medical contract for which it is meant. In gene technology we have access to forces which, if not controlled and regulated, can create unexpected and unpredictable situations.

Preparation of transgene animals. The food and pharmaceutical industries may express strong interest in producing so-called transgene animals, in which genes are transferred between different species. This can make it possible to adjust the meat to the needs of human beings. But there are cases of this which cause the animals a great deal of suffering. For example, pigs who have received genes from strange species have been deformed; they suffer difficulties in breathing, bad eyesight and high sensitivity to infections. Such gene transformation can also be regarded as a definite violation of the dignity and integrity of the biological community.

If the preparation of transgene animals involves a violation of and suffering for the animals, we believe such preparation should be forbidden. When it comes to preparation of transgene animals for food production, the prohibition must be without exception. Such a preparation implies a violation of the intrinsic value of animals. To counter the argument that such a prohibition will increase the importation of such meat from places where it is permitted, we think there should also be a ban on such imports or a requirement that meat from transgene animals must be clearly indicated as such.

When it comes to preparation of transgene animals for research and production of medicine, our basic position is the same. But we recognize that there are important additional elements in this case. New knowledge which is not available elsewhere may be gained through such research. The production of certain medicines may become less expensive and safer. So we believe the preparation of transgene animals for research and production of medicines is acceptable *during a transitional stage*, provided that the animals do not suffer and that there is no alternative way to gain this knowledge or produce these medicines. While a violation of the animals' integrity is involved, we believe that this violation, under the conditions mentioned, must be considered well-motivated. By using the term "transitional stage", we want to emphasize that in the long run other ways should be found to reach the specific aim.

Some would assert that the preparation of transgene animals for food production is a question of human survival. But this is not the case presently. That is why the ethical question has to be raised continuously. On the one hand, the Christian faith teaches that human beings are mandated to administer the created world and to use nature and its resources for the survival of humanity. On the other hand, human beings are to exercise this management gently and in a way that does not irrevocably damage nature. Human beings do not have the right to cause suffering to their fellow human beings or other creatures.

Transplantation of tissue from an aborted foetus. The question of whether it is generally permissible to transplant tissue from aborted foetuses has been given topical interest by experiments to cure people who are suffering from Parkinson's disease and diabetes. It is agreed in this context that (1) it is always good to want to cure sick people, (2) aborted foetuses are readily available and the tissue of these foetuses will be wasted if it is not used, and (3) that the meaninglessness of the fate of aborted foetuses is transformed into meaning when they become of use for other people as "organ donors".

There is no doubt that curing diseases is a good action. Christian theology has seen healing as part of the struggle against the evil in life and a consequence of the gospel. According to the New Testament, Jesus sent his disciples in order to preach the gospel and to cure sick people. But the fact that the curing of diseases is a good action does not mean that it may be done at any price. There is still the limit set by the integrity of the fellow-being. A foetus also has this dignity and integrity; and an aborted foetus should be shown the same respect and consideration as any dead human being who could possibly be an organ donor. Since the church considers a foetus as a human life, the same rule must be applied to the foetus as in the case of a minor: informed consent must be given by the mother before the organ to be transplanted can be taken.

This consensus has not been questioned, with a few exceptions, in the debate: it has been considered natural that the woman should decide whether or not her aborted foetus is to become an organ donor. Yet a woman who is considering abortion is hardly free in the sense of giving this consent. She is at a disadvantage, and it is quite possible that she may feel that she is forced to consent to the donation of tissue from the foetus.

It is well known that organ transplants from a close relative are more likely to be successful than transplants from unrelated people. Thus one can imagine a scenario in which a young woman is persuaded to get pregnant and then have an abortion in order to provide foetal tissue for a grandparent suffering from Parkinson's disease or diabetes. This possibility, which is not far-fetched, illustrates the obvious risk of objectifying the foetus and reducing human life to a remedy for someone else. We do not know to what extent the taking of organs from aborted foetuses may influence the rate of abortion and the demand for aborted foetuses. At present, three or four foetuses are needed to treat one patient. Perhaps this may decrease in the future. But at the same time the number of new fields of application might increase considerably. Thus we regard an established activity of transplanting tissue from aborted foetuses as the beginning of a slippery slope.

The fact that we advise against transplantation of tissue from aborted foetuses and see such activity as violating human value does not mean that we do not care about finding a remedy for Parkinson's disease and other diseases that medical science tries to cure in this way. But we do not see the only alternatives as transplantation and passive acceptance of the diseases. Experiments to find remedies through cell-culture have been done, and this research should be supported and developed.

* * *

In this letter we have tried to explain that science and technical development, according to the Christian view of creation and the human being, are considered positively, but that there are limits which this activity must not and cannot exceed without violating the integrity of human beings and creation.

From a Christian point of view, the dignity and integrity of human beings must not be violated, and the integrity of the rest of creation may be violated only in very exceptional cases. The three concrete examples we have addressed may leave the impression that the church wants to forbid or at least strongly limit biotechnology. That is not the case. The three examples point to the limits that cannot be exceeded without transforming the human being into an object and reducing it to a remedy for the comfort of another or causing animals manipulation and suffering. But we have also identified the possibility of going beyond these limits in clearly motivated cases.

We as Christians see large possibilities in biotechnology as well. It can, if correctly developed, become a great asset to human beings and their environment. We have already mentioned the production of medicines. A problem in this connection is that this research has concentrated on the needs of people in the West, where there are already good medicines in many cases, while virtually ignoring the need for medicines and vaccines in the economically poorer parts of the world. Through biotechnology it might be possible to increase the grain crop in order to improve the food supply in the world. There are also hopes that certain types of environmental pollution may be taken care of by biotechnology. There are many other possible future applications of biotechnology; the problem is again that it is often economic profitability that has a disproportionate influence on how biotechnology companies choose to focus their activity.

We wish you joy and blessing in your work as a parliamentarian, and we hope that this letter will help you to make decisions when legislation on biotechnology and how it should be applied to human beings, animals and vegetables is discussed. As a politician you have a very important task in stimulating people to find new medicines, technologies and methods of treatment. But you also have a very important task in regulating and legislating for medicine and science in order to respect and preserve human dignity and the integrity of the creation.

Greetings,
From your congregation

9. *Ethics and Counselling*

A Letter to a Fellow Pastor

SVEIN AAGE CHRISTOFFERSEN
and VIGGO MORTENSEN

Dear George,

It was a pleasant surprise to hear from you after so long. I still cherish the memory of the years we spent together at the seminary and the intense discussions we used to have about theology. I gather from your letter that you rarely find the time these days to delve deeply into theological reflection the way we did then. I still find it rewarding to take time for that kind of reflection, and I would encourage you to do the same.

As to the question of bioethics, which you raise in your letter, I would say that it is virtually a duty of the church to keep the discussion of these issues alive — though I can sympathize with your somewhat sarcastic reference to the "flood" of talk about ethics that comes from every quarter these days. At times I find it frustrating to relate to the constant demand for "ethics" from politicians, administrators, business people, journalists and others. One has the impression that some of these people have no idea what they are asking for, while others simply want concrete answers and guidelines without having to bother with the reasoning that leads to such conclusions. As we learned in the seminary long ago, ethics is not like that. You cannot just copy a conclusion in ethics without at least a tentative understanding of why this is a possible conclusion and what arguments can be raised against it. But when you tell people that in ethics there is no easy way out, that you have to engage yourself in the ethical discourse, many of them lose interest.

Another problem is that ethics often seems to come in too late in the game, only after something has gone wrong. It is a substitute for the good life which should have flourished. In other words, ethics lives from something "pre-ethical" — an inspiring vision of the good life, whether it comes from the Bible, or from the arts and culture or from the struggle of the people.

But I nevertheless agree with you that we cannot let these difficulties discourage us from promoting and encouraging bioethical discourse within the church as well as in society at large. My own impression is that public discourse on this subject is in great danger of becoming "homeless". There are plenty of arenas today where bioethical questions can be the subject of confrontations and battles — talk shows on television and radio, editorials and letters to the editor in newspapers and magazines and of course in chambers and corridors of legislatures. But it is very often the case in these arenas that economic interests play the major role behind the points of view being advanced. What we need today is a place where it is permitted not to be absolutely certain, a place for questioning and listening, for raising doubts and hesitation, for thinking and rethinking — a place where ordinary people can address bioethical questions from their own point of view. We need a space where bioethical questions can be considered, debated and discussed, not just fought over. It seems to me that the church could be such a place. I think it is of vital importance that the church not just act as a pressure group on bioethics but also serve as a host for bioethical deliberation.

Your letter makes the important point that bioethical questions are closely connected to the core of Christian faith and at the same time of vital concern to many of the ordinary members of the church. Every pastor who cares about his or her congregation will in one way or another be confronted with bioethical questions, and they should be addressed in adult education, pastoral care and from the pulpit. While I agree fully with this, I think it is important for pastors to bear in mind when addressing bioethical questions that their main task is to proclaim the gospel. A pastor is not a legislator or judge or professional moralizer, but a herald of God's unlimited grace in Jesus Christ.

Here I think that we as Christians have a definite advantage. Without being "foundationalist" or "fundamentalist", we do have something to build upon. It is found in the biblical text and the

Christian tradition. This foundation is at the same time radical and not always concrete. But then we also have a story — the stories Jesus told and the stories told about him. All of this is handed down to us through texts which bear witness to the fact that the basic questions about being a human person have been dealt with before. When we make this story our own, the texts help us to be more attentive to moral dilemmas and force us to look in a specific direction. In Christian ethics there is always a preferential option for the weaker party. This is enjoined in the great commandment: love God above all and your neighbour as yourself. This radical commandment should be responded to in accordance with the person Jesus. Even if we can never fully imitate Christ, who was the Son of God, we have in him an example that will always keep us honest. In him we see an attitude of compassion incarnate, which can also be a directive for us whenever we try to make our choices and live our lives to the glory of God and the benefit of our neighbour.

Bioethical questions are often questions people have to answer for themselves. A pastor's task is not to tell people what they have to do, but to help them to take decisions of their own which they can identify themselves with in years to come. You are right in saying that society and technology place heavy burdens on people's shoulders these days. They have to make decisions about life and death in situations that were unknown even a couple of decades ago. Sometimes I think these burdens are too heavy, and that we must somehow change society to spare people decisions like these. But that is probably a utopian thought; and in any case we may not simply ignore all the people who do have to take a decision here and now.

To say that people must take a decision of their own, not just choose whatever they think is expected of them, does not mean taking a decision *alone*. On the contrary, one needs the help and support of other people if one is to decide freely. That is the paradox of freedom.

An aspect of decision-making that is often forgotten is the importance of a long-term perspective. The question is not only what is most convenient to do here and now, but also what kind of decision one will be able to live with in years to come. Since choices have to be made, it is of vital importance that we as pastors help people to live with their choices. Some will regret their choices afterwards; others will be haunted by doubts and uncertainty; still others will remain convinced of their choice but still have to live with difficult and perhaps painful consequences. A decision on a difficult bioethical question is not the end, but the beginning of a new phase in which a person must struggle with new questions from another angle. Perhaps the notion of the forgiveness of sins can take on new importance under these circumstances.

After several years of more or less constantly discussing bioethical questions, publicly as well as privately, I have concluded that one of the most important things a pastor can do is to *listen* — to members of the congregation who come asking for advice or just looking for someone to talk to, to doctors, nurses and researchers when they present their dilemmas. Unfortunately, many people today have lost faith in the pastor as a person who is able to listen. Through the centuries the church has built up the image of a pastor as a man (yes, a *man*!) whose primary task is to issue statements and give orders. This role must be changed. Out of genuine love we as pastors need to stand by the people who are dealing with life-and-death issues.

Well, these have been some random observations in response to some of the issues you mention in your letter. The bottom line is that I think that one of the most important things we learned at the seminary still holds true: we need to base our thinking on a Christian view of what it is to be a human being. No man or woman is an island. We live as parts of other people's lives, as they are parts of our lives. We have to preserve and nurture this inter-relatedness. Biotechnology can be used to sort people out, to get rid of those who are different, differently abled. But that would be terribly wrong, and we cannot accept that kind of society. On the contrary, as pastors we must advocate for a caring society; and I think you are right to suggest that we ought to get together more regularly to prepare ourselves to face these challenges.

Why don't we both ask around about the interest among our colleagues in forming a small group to do this kind of reflection and discussion? I think we need to find the right mixture of pastors and men and women from other professions. But we can discuss the composition of the group in more detail later. Until then, I send you my best wishes and look forward to hearing from you further.

Sincerely yours,
Peter

10. *Mandatory Genetic Testing*

A Letter to the Manager of a Pharmaceutical Company

SAKARI KARJALAINEN
and ULLA SCHMIDT

Dear Mr Larson,

We have learned that your company is seriously considering the introduction of gene testing of all employees. As we understand it, this is meant to be compulsory for all workers and probably all future job-applicants.

This measure could seriously affect many of your employees, both on the job and in their personal, social and economic life. So we believe that it is of utmost importance to consider this issue very carefully in terms of the fundamental and critical ethical problems it raises.

The context of our concerns is our own Lutheran tradition, which determines and conditions our perspective. In particular we would emphasize the weight given within the Lutheran tradition to the notion of natural law and such basic principles embodied in it as fundamental human dignity and the right to life. These principles are in conformity with such specifically Christian principles as neighbourly love and the Golden Rule, which are further specified in more concrete principles like justice, equality, beneficence, autonomy and liberty — all of them of great relevance for the issues at stake here.

Given the importance of the notion of vocation in Lutheran ethics, one of our main concerns is to consider the important principles and concerns which characterize your own role and function as the manager of this company. One way in which we think that you may fruitfully approach the topic is to consider what weight you as a manager ought to give to various interests in assessing the proposal of gene-testing. You might argue that your major concern and responsibility, to which all other concerns should be subjected, is the total health of the company, especially as measured by its economic results. By putting the effectiveness and profit of the company first, you could claim, you are in fact acting in the best way you can to fulfil your responsibility to your employees. However important and legitimate this interest, we want to suggest that there are others as well which need to be taken into account by the manager of a company like yours.

Genetic testing: why and how?

To investigate ethically the measure you are planning, it might be useful to begin by looking more closely at the background of this proposal. What purposes is it supposed to serve, and what means are employed to achieve them?

First, the most obvious reason seems to be avoiding unnecessary risk for employees. Needless to say, any working situation implies various kinds of risks for the employees, ranging from exposure to radiation and contact with chemicals and toxic waste to things like noise and stress. Some of these risks involve accidents like explosions or instantaneous poisoning; others have to do with exposure over many years which may lead to certain illnesses — like the risk of developing cancer from exposure to certain kinds of radiation. Obviously, a company and its managers have a primary responsibility to minimize risks, but in certain industries it may be impossible to eliminate the risk totally.

It may be that not all employees are equally susceptible to some of these risks, but that the danger either arises or increases considerably for persons of a certain genetic makeup, which predisposes them to certain illnesses. Two employees in the same working situations thus might run very dissimilar risks; likewise a person might have very different chances of developing an illness depending on the conditions he or she is working under, if that person has a particular genetic disposition. For example, a worker with a genetic predisposition to develop certain types of cancer is probably much more at risk if exposed to radiation on the job than if he or she had a different kind of job. Thus one method to avoid or at least minimize risks of this type is to test employees genetically for such disorders and remove them if necessary from high-risk situations.

But a second, perhaps related reason for introducing this measure could be not merely to protect workers from risks, but also to avoid hiring people with features supposed to disqualify them for the work. Genetic tests would be one more in a series of tests and evaluations used for selecting employees.

Gene-testing raises a further problem related to the methods. Whether for purposes of security or selection, there is always a problem with projects of sampling and registering data of a personal character, whether it is done by way of genetic testing or other means. The risk is always present that the information, even though collected for a justifiable purpose, is not sufficiently safeguarded against wrongful use of various kinds. The more intimate and private this information, the greater the potential harm to the persons surveyed.

Three ethical principles

When we ask whether gene-testing is an ethically viable option, certain fundamental ethical principles come into play. These principles serve as a normative basis and provide a perspective for considering the specific issue, as it is presumably these principles which are especially threatened by this option. Part of your responsibility might thus be to acknowledge and act on the fundamental role played by these principles within our ethical tradition.

The principle of autonomy. The individual has a fundamental right to determine and decide about his own life; and it would usually be a breach of the principle of autonomy for someone else to take control in an important respect over a person's life, ordering or even forcing him or her to do this or that. Any kind of illegal coercion of a person against his or her will would be a violation of the principle of autonomy. But it is important here to notice the sense in which we are talking about autonomy. The function of the right to autonomy as applied here is to protect the individual from wrongful mistreatment, abuse, interference and so forth (in other words, negative rights), not primarily to ensure the right to pursue one's own goals, wishes, purposes (in the sense of positive rights, as claimed most notably within the libertarian tradition).

Thus the right to autonomy is adequately interpreted as an instrument for pursuing and safeguarding the content of the Golden Rule and beneficence. It protects important aspects of human life and dignity. There might be cases of restrictions on autonomy, for example where persons cannot be assumed to know what is best for them, but this restraint will then be in need of a further justification of itself, which could override the autonomy-principle. These should be strong reasons, as the principle of autonomy is taken to be fundamental, safeguarding values we usually consider as highly important for the possibility of a good human life. It protects persons from wrongful coercion and victimization of several kinds, leaving them with a fundamental responsibility for and freedom of their own lives, which seems to be inherently connected to our conception of human dignity. One implication of this principle would be the right to privacy, that is the right to have a personal sphere in which no one else is permitted to interfere without a person's consent.

The principle of beneficence. One situation in which autonomy would legitimately be restricted is where it conflicts with the principle of beneficence. This principle states that wherever it is in one's power and knowledge to do so, one always has a duty to seek to do good to people rather than evil. If I am able to benefit another person presumably in need of help, I ought to do so. A weaker version of the principle merely says I should always avoid harming someone. Obviously, the principles of autonomy and beneficence can easily run into conflict, for example, when a person is about to do something (as an expression of his or her legitimate autonomy) which I know would lead to harmful consequences for him or her. This is why children and persons who are mentally ill, for example, have only a very restricted autonomy, as they cannot be expected to know what is truly for their best. But problems arise when people know (or claim to know) what is best for other adults, and so believe that they may rightly infringe on their autonomy in the name of beneficence. Which principle should be assigned greater weight is in many cases not at all clear.

The principle of justice. A third relevant ethical principle offering a fruitful perspective on the issue is the principle of justice. Justice has been defined in many different ways, but one simple way of articulating it is in terms of a duty not to discriminate against anyone for irrelevant reasons. Fundamentally, everyone has a right to a fair equality in opportunities, for the satisfaction of legitimate needs, education, work and so on. No one should be denied equality of opportunity except for relevant reasons. Similarly no unreasonably heavy burden (for example, economically) should be laid on anyone except for relevant reasons. Consequently, to justify treating two persons differently in the same area (for example, in the allocation of resources), one must be able to point to a *relevant* difference between them.

Problems with genetic testing

Genetic testing and risk-protection. We noted earlier that the most important reason for introducing genetic testing is to protect workers from unnecessary and unknown risks. By detecting the genetic disposition to certain illnesses, the employer can move the employee to another kind of work so as to avoid or minimize the risk.

Since this would obviously be for the benefit of employees with such a disposition, it might seem to be a justifiable and viable way of complying with your fundamental responsibility for the well-being of your employees. We assume that the company has already undertaken all possible efforts to make the working place as clean and safe as possible for the protection of the labourers, and that the idea of gene-testing is to introduce protection of a secondary kind. As a means of minimizing the risk to employees of developing a serious illness, genetic testing would respond to their fundamental right to a life without unnecessary pain and suffering, which underlies the principle of beneficence.

Our main objection is to making this testing mandatory for all employees. The employee is thus required and obliged to give away information about his or her genetic structure and dispositions. We believe this might violate another fundamental interest and right of the employee which you should take into account. How this might be an infringement of fundamental rights can be spelled out along two lines. First, the fundamental right of autonomy (especially formulated as the right to privacy) includes the right not to be forced to reveal personal and intimate information about oneself. It is evident that this right could be overridden if the absence of such information implied danger or harm to someone else, but that is not the case here. Second, this right to privacy would seem to imply a right *not* to be informed about one's genetic disorders against one's own wish, that is, a right to remain uninformed. A person may well believe that ignorance about whether or not he or she carries a genetic disposition for some ailment makes it more likely that he or she can enjoy a good life. This right to make this deliberate choice for ignorance might be undermined by this measure, for example, if a worker suddenly finds himself or herself removed from his or her usual job. The possibility of unexpected findings through these tests, which would probably be revealed to the employee, should also be taken into account.

But, you may object, the test may benefit the employee greatly anyway. Should this not count as an argument for overriding a person's autonomy in the name of providing good for him or her? However, assuming that the employees have been fully and sufficiently informed about the risks and dangers they may be exposed to at work, as well as about the specific risk to those who carry a special genetic disorder, there can be no reason to assume that the employee is not capable of making a reasonable and right judgment about what is for his or her own best in this situation. If the employee is fully aware of the facts and still thinks it for the best not to reveal or to be informed about his or her genetic status, there is no justification for forcing a test. To be sure, an employer is justified in many respects in obliging workers to comply with various security measures without admitting any choice or reservation on the part of the employee — the wearing of helmets or protective clothing or safety belts for example. But we would argue that such measures do not interfere with the personal and private sphere in the same way that a genetic test does. They do not breach the right of autonomy. Consequently, we would strongly argue that genetic testing should be *offered to* employees, but by no means *forced on* anyone. The explicit consent of the employee to undergo the test should always be required.

Moreover, if the purpose of the test is to protect the workers from certain work-related risks, there should probably be a differentiation, designing separate tests according to the risk connected with each specific working situation. It is apparent that not all employees are exposed to similar risks; and since information collected by the company should be directly relevant to the purpose for which it is collected, employees in different departments should undergo different tests.

Furthermore, the seriousness of the risk — how great a risk for how serious an ailment — should be weighed against the unease of the prospect of changing jobs. In certain situations, the latter possibility might cause great personal economic and social difficulties. An employee may not consider the risk to be serious enough to warrant changing jobs, or perhaps even face the possibility of being laid off if the company cannot offer him another job. In this situation, too, we believe the employee should have the final word. If he or she prefers a less safe job to no job at all, or to great difficulties of other kinds, that choice should be accepted, provided that he or she has been adequately and sufficiently informed. Thus gene tests should not be forced on employees.

A difficult situation arises when an applicant agrees to undergo a test, and a disorder implying high risk of developing a certain illness, directly related to the job in question, is detected. Would you as an employer be justified in denying the applicant the job on this condition, on the ground that it involves too great a risk for the person, even though the applicant himself or herself does not withdraw the application? Admittedly, this is an unusual and awkward situation: why would an applicant, after consenting to the test, refuse to take the precautions suggested by its results? It seems to us that the company might be justified in not hiring the applicant in such a case. What you are not justified in doing, however, is forcing the test on him or her.

Genetic testing and selection of workers. We said earlier that your role as a manager includes a fundamental, legitimate and important responsibility for the company's productivity, effectiveness and profit. This is not in itself governed by selfish or "illegitimate" interests, for it is likely to benefit your employees and society as a whole if this responsibility is carefully fulfilled. To ensure the improvement of the economic situation of the company and secure its financial soundness and stability, it is necessary to select the most skilled and qualified workers available for various jobs in the company. A company is therefore justified in applying different means to test its employees and applicants. So it might also be in the company's interest to avoid hiring persons with certain genetic dispositions (for example, to develop certain illnesses) or with certain permanent weaknesses of a psychological or mental character, which would decrease their performance as workers, even though this is not related to any specific condition in the work itself. Could genetic testing for this purpose be justified?

Here, too, the fundamental principles of autonomy and beneficence of course come into play. And again, we find it highly doubtful that the principle of autonomy — in the specific form of the principle of privacy (that one should not be forced to reveal personal and intimate information about oneself without relevant reasons) — may be overridden by the interest of the company in selecting the most suitable and skilled employees. The principle of autonomy seems to be safeguarding values of human life which are more fundamental than the right to seek profit and effectiveness, even though the latter is a legitimate value and interest.

The case becomes even more doubtful if the testing is done not only in order to select the most skilled applicant in a group of applicants for a job, but also in order to select for dismissal employees with "disapproved" qualities in genetic terms (for instance, in a situation when it is necessary to decrease the work-force). Indeed, this would not comply with the principle of beneficence, even in its weaker form of avoiding harm, as it would impose severe harm on the employee.

You might object that in such a situation harm will be imposed on employees anyway: someone will be selected for the job and others will not; some people will be laid off in economic bad times and others will keep their job. It is impossible completely to avoid bringing about harm to any employees or applicants. Our question, then, is whether the harm is being distributed according to relevant criteria. In the situation we are describing it is obviously distributed in relation to the genetic disposition of the respective employees. Quite apart from the question of whether it is justifiable to require such information from applicants or employees at all, is discrimination in this respect justifiable or not? It is our opinion that it can hardly be regarded as a relevant reason for discrimination that a person is disposed to or carries the risk of developing a certain malady presumably years from now. Moreover, one may question whether it is a sufficient justification for discriminating against certain employees to refer to circumstances which they have not chosen or had a fair opportunity to choose for themselves.

Persons with certain disabilities, especially those over which they themselves have no control, should be granted fair equality of opportunity, along with other persons. This would seem especially important in cases where persons with certain dispositions would be hindered in or even denied access to the work-force in general, as might happen if genetic testing is done more commonly. The standards according to which employees are selected for gene-tests may also be unclear. If the purpose is to discover features that are definitely disabling for a given job, these could presumably be discovered by other means as well. Moreover, the boundary between "disability" in this strong sense and capacities or features which are merely undesirable for some reason is not all that clear, but the latter do not serve as a sufficient criterion for selection and access to work.

Furthermore, your responsibility for the well-being of the employees within their working situation can also be linked to the more basic roles that having a job and doing work are assigned within human life — serving other people and society in general, self-realization, a sense of accomplishment at overcoming challenges and solving problems. In general, having a job contributes to our possibility of leading a good life. These important aspects of the role of being an employee ought also to be acknowledged and safeguarded by the company and its management. We would want to claim that a part of your responsibility as a manager is to ensure that the possibility for your employees to experience their work in this way is not undermined but promoted and enhanced (which in turn may contribute to a rise in the company's productivity and profit). But it is exactly this which risks being undermined by the introduction of mandatory gene-testing. Being tested with respect to such natural or biological characteristics and capacities is quite different from being tested for other types of compliance with the standards of the job. There seems to be a qualitative difference between subjecting employees to this kind of genetic screening and testing with respect to how well or poorly they accomplish their work in general. The latter may easily be compatible with your fundamental responsibility for the workers, whereas the former seems not to be.

Thus we believe that the introduction of predictive gene testing for the purpose of selection on the basis of suitability for the job in general would breach important principles of justice and imply an unjust treatment of some persons in the sense of discriminating against them on the basis of irrelevant characteristics.

Genetic testing and data-registration. Finally, we want to draw your attention briefly to another obvious ethical problem arising from the means employed in gene testing. Presumably, what you intend to do is not only to test the employees, but also to collect and record this information, which is of a very sensitive and intimate kind, in an efficient way. Three problems should be indicated here:

1. With any type of data-processing, there is always the chance that the data thus collected and stored are actually wrong. And when these data are to be used for such far-reaching decisions as here, this risk should not be underestimated. This risk can of course be diminished, but it cannot be eliminated entirely.

2. There is always a risk that data stored in a register will be used, without the consent of the informant, for a purpose other than what they were originally sampled for. As the information in this case is of a highly personal character, such use would be unacceptable, and the existence of such a risk would be an argument against the storage of information of this kind.

3. Obviously there is also a risk that the protection of confidentiality of the information is not sufficient, so that other persons or groups may gain access to the data without the knowledge and consent of the person concerned.

* * *

In drawing this letter to a close we want to emphasize again that if the company is to introduce gene-testing for the employees, it should not be mandatory. The final decision should always be left to each employee, and he or she should not be subjected to any kind of direct or indirect pressure to consent to it. Only in this way can important values applying to fundamental dimensions of human dignity, like autonomy and the right to privacy, protection from unnecessary harm and the right to just treatment be safeguarded and promoted. As we have said, we believe that these interests and values are an integral part of your primary responsibility as a manager to your employees. Moreover, such testing should be applied only for the purpose of protection against risks which cannot be eliminated by other measures. And the risks pertaining to the registration of such information should be specifically acknowledged and addressed.

Yours sincerely,
J.-P. Williams
(on behalf of concerned staff)

Contributors

Svend Andersen, Evangelical Lutheran Church in Denmark. He is professor of ethics and philosophy of religion at the University of Aarhus.

Björn Björnsson, Evangelical Lutheran Church in Iceland. He is professor of ethics at the University of Iceland.

Svein Aage Christoffersen, Church of Norway. He is professor of systematic theology, University of Oslo.

Jaana Hallamaa, Evangelical Lutheran Church of Finland. She is associate professor of systematic theology at the University of Helsinki.

Jukka-Mikko Karjalainen, Evangelical Lutheran Church of Finland. He is a pastor in Vantaa, Finland.

Sakari Karjalainen, Evangelical Lutheran Church of Finland. He is a medical doctor and secretary general of the Medical Research Council of Finland (Academy of Finland), Helsinki.

Lena Kjems, Evangelical Lutheran Church in Denmark. She is a doctoral student at the Centre for Bioethics of the University of Aarhus.

Kees van Kooten Niekerk, Reformed. He is senior research associate at the Centre for Bioethics at the University of Aarhus.

Hans-Olof Kvist, Evangelical Lutheran Church of Finland. He is professor of systematic theology at the Theological Faculty, Åbo Akademi University.

Viggo Mortensen, Evangelical Lutheran Church in Denmark. He is director, Department for Theology and Studies, and secretary for the Church and Social Issues, Lutheran World Federation, Geneva, Switzerland.

Gert Nilsson, Church of Sweden. He is docent for ethics and systematic theology in the Research Department of the Church of Sweden, Uppsala.

Lars Østnor, Church of Norway. He is professor of systematic theology at the Norwegian Lutheran School of Theology, Oslo.

Ulla Schmidt, Church of Norway. She is a doctoral student in ethics at the Norwegian Lutheran School of Theology, Oslo.

Per Sundström, Church of Sweden. He is a researcher at the University of Uppsala, Sweden.

Anne-Marie Thunberg, Church of Sweden. She is an ethicist and editor in Sigtuna, Sweden.

Lars Thunberg, Church of Sweden. He is former associate professor of systematic theology at the Universities of Uppsala and Aarhus.